Viva Voce in

Experimental Pharmacology

for Undergraduate and Postgraduate Students

Viva Voce in

Experimental Pharmacology

for Undergraduate and Postgraduate Students

Amteshwar Singh Jaggi
M Pharm, PhD (Pharmacology)

Assistant Professor in Pharmacology
Department of Pharmaceutical Sciences and
Drug Research, Patiala, Punjab

Anjana Bali
M Pharm (Pharmacology)

Senior Research Fellow (DST)
Department of Pharmaceutical Sciences and
Drug Research, Patiala, Punjab

Nirmal Singh
M Pharm PhD (Pharmacology)

Associate Professor in Pharmacology
Department of Pharmaceutical Sciences and
Drug Research, Patiala, Punjab

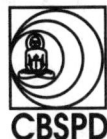

CBSPD

CBS Publishers & Distributors Pvt Ltd

New Delhi • Bengaluru • Chennai • Kochi • Kolkata • Lucknow• Mumbai
Hyderabad • Jharkhand • Nagpur • Patna • Pune • Uttarakhand

Viva Voce in
Experimental Pharmacology

ISBN: 978-81-239-2520-2

Copyright © Authors and Publisher

First Edition: 2015
Reprint: 2018, 2019, 2020, 2024

Published by Satish Kumar Jain and produced by Varun Jain for
CBS Publishers & Distributors Pvt Ltd
4819/XI Prahlad Street, 24 Ansari Road, Daryaganj, New Delhi 110 002, India.
Ph: 23289259, 23266861   Website: www.cbspd.com
                              e-mail: delhi@cbspd.com
Corporate Office: 204 FIE, Industrial Area, Patparganj, Delhi 110 092
Ph: 011-4934 4934   Fax: 011-4934 4935   e-mail: publishing@cbspd.com;
                                             publicity@cbspd.com

Branches

- **Bengaluru:** Seema House 2975, 17th Cross, K.R. Road, Banasankari 2nd Stage,
  Bengaluru 560 070, Karnataka
  Ph: +91-80-26771678/79   Fax: +91-80-26771680   e-mail: bangalore@cbspd.com
- **Chennai:** 7, Subbaraya Street, Shenoy Nagar, Chennai 600 030, Tamil Nadu, India
  Ph: +91-44-26680620/26681266   Fax: +91-44-42032115   e-mail: chennai@cbspd.com
- **Kochi:** 42/1325, 1326, Power House Road, Opp KSEB, Power House, Ernakulam 682 018,
  Kochi, Kerala, India
  Ph: +91-484-4059061-65, 67   Fax: +91-484-4059065   e-mail: kochi@cbspd.com
- **Kolkata:** 147, Hind Ceramics Compound, 1st Floor, Nilgunj Road, Belghoria, Kolkata-700056,
  West Bengal, India
  Ph: +033-25633055, 033-25633056   e-mail: kolkata@cbspd.com
- **Lucknow:** Basement, Khushnuma Complex, 7 Meerabai Marg (Behind Jawahar Bhawan),
  Lucknow-226001, UP, India
  Ph: +91-522-4000032   e-mail: tiwari.lucknow@cbspd.com
- **Mumbai:** PWD Shed, Gala no 25/26, Ramchandra Bhatt Marg, Next to JJ Hospital
  Gate no. 2, Opp. Union Bank of India Noorbaug, Mumbai-400009, Maharashtra, India
  Ph: 022-66661880/89   e-mail: mumbai@cbspd.com

Representatives

- **Hyderabad**   U-9885175004   - **Jharkhand**   0 9811641605   - **Nagpur**   0-8692091830
- **Patna**   0-9334159340   - **Pune**   0-9664372571   - **Uttarakhand** 0-9716462459

Printed at: SRK Graphics, Shahdara, Delhi, India

to

our loving families

Preface

The field of pharmacology is expanding at a tremendous rate and new drugs are being developed very briskly. Since the discovery and evaluation of new drugs depend on the platform of good experimental designing of pharmacology experiments, it is utmost necessary for the students of pharmacology (and even non-pharmacology students) to understand the basic aspects of experimental pharmacology. The present book attempts to clarify the basic aspects of experimental pharmacology in the form of questions and answers. The book is meant for both undergraduates and postgraduates, and each chapter is divided into two sections for the same purpose. The key feature of this book is the choice of animal species for a particular disease model, i.e. which animal species is particularly important for inducing a particular disease. The ethical issues related to animal usage and common basic questions related to application of statistics in pharmacology are the core features of this book. Furthermore, the chapters related to experimental designing, toxicity studies and bioassay are also incorporated.

Nevertheless, the main emphasis is laid on the conventional *in vitro* experiments (DRC-related) and *in vivo* disease model-related experiments. We hope that the book shall cater to the needs of undergraduate as well as postgraduate students and even young faculty in understanding the basic aspects related to common pharmacology experiments.

Amteshwar Singh Jaggi
Anjana Bali
Nirmal Singh

Acknowledgments

Everybody makes an attempt to achieve success. However, only those become successful for whom God makes an effort. This project is solely due to God's effort and authors thank the Almighty for providing us the energy to put the efforts and also paveing the way for its successful completion.

We wish to acknowledge Department of Pharmaceutical Sciences and Drug Research, Punjabi University, Patiala, for providing us the platform and technical facilities for this project. We wish to thank all our colleagues, friends, and well-wishers of our department who directly or indirectly provided the support and motivation continuously. We wish to acknowledge our pharmacology teachers of this department Late Prof Manjeet Singh and Dr. Ajay Sharma who have contributed in understanding the basic fundamentals of pharmacology. We wish to thank our students (particularly research scholars) who contributed in better understanding of this matter. We particularly want to acknowledge Ms Puneet Kaur Randhawa for helping us in final editing of this book.

Family is the main pillar which provides us the actual support, makes us thrive and stand with us all the time. The authors wish to acknowledge their family members and friends (like a family member) S. Narinder Singh Jaggi, Smt Harvinder Kaur, Late S. Gurbax Singh Anand, Smt Rajinder Kaur Anand, Dr Jaspal Kaur, Dr Preet Jaggi, Brahmjagteshwar Singh, Sarbeshwar Kaur Jaggi, Mrs Neetu, Aryan Puru, Mr Ram Lal Bali, Smt Jasvir Kaur, Mr Jagdish Rai, Smt Surinder Kaur, Mr Ashok Kumar Bali, Mrs Rajwant Kaur, Mrs Renu, Mr Jasvir Singh, Mr Vippen Bali, Rippen, Jasmine, Sameer, Ms Monika Rani and Mr Sikander Garg.

Last but not the least, we beg forgiveness of all those who have been with us over the years and whose names we have failed to mention.

Amteshwar Singh Jaggi
Anjana Bali
Nirmal Singh

Contents

Type of Animals Employed in Experimental Pharmacology

FOR UNDERGRADUATES AND POSTGRADUATES

1. **Classify experimental animals employed in pharmacology.**

Ans: Experimental animals are mainly divided into three categories:

Rodents: Mouse, rat, Guinea pig, gerbil, hamster, etc. (Fig. 1.1)

Non-rodents: Rabbit, monkey, dog, cat, pig

Miscellaneous: Pigeon, frog, etc.

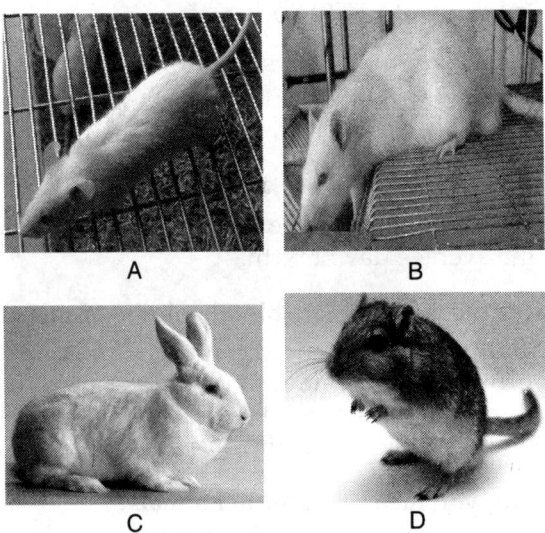

Fig. 1.1: Commonly employed animals in experimental pharmacology
A—mouse; B—rat; C—rabbit; D—hamster

2. **What are the most commonly used animals in experimental pharmacological research?**

Ans: Mice are the most commonly employed animals in experimental research followed by rats. These account for 90% of the mammals used for research.

3. **Why are these animals very commonly employed?**

Ans: These animals are very commonly employed due to following reasons:
   a. These are very well characterized anatomically, physiologically and genetically.
   b. These are resilient, adaptable, easy to care, handle, inexpensive.
   c. Due to their small size, these can be housed in large numbers.
   d. They have short generation time and high reproductive potential.
   e. The results obtained from these can be translated to good extent to humans.

4. **What is the average lifespan of rats or mice?**

Ans: Average lifespan of rats or mice is 2–4 years and 1.5–3 years, respectively.

5. **What is the reproductive stage of rats?**

Ans: The average reproductive stage of rats starts from 8 to 10 weeks.

6. **What is the gestation period of rats?**

Ans: The average gestation period is 21–23 days and 22nd day is the average day of birth.

7. **What is the approximate blood volume of rats and mice?**

Ans: The approximate blood volume of adult mice is 2.25 ml approx., for 25 gm mouse (90 ml/kg of body weight) and for rats, it is around 16 ml approx. for 250 gm rat (64 ml/kg of body weight).

8. **What do you mean by albino animals?**

Ans: Albino means colorless and these are white due to absence of melanin. Albino refers to animals that completely lack the pigmentation.

9. What are the most commonly employed strains of rats in pharmacology?

Ans: Wistar and Sprague Dawley rats are the most commonly employed strains of rats in pharmacology.

10. Why are Wistar rats so called?

Ans: The Wistar rats are named after the "Wistar Institute of Anatomy and Biology in Philadelphia" where the Wistar stock of *Rattus norvegicus* (scientific name of Norway rats) was established. It is characterized by its wide head, long ears, and has a tail length that is always less than its body length.

11. What is Sprague Dawley rat?

Ans: This strain has been developed from Wistar rats and this breed of rat was first produced by the Sprague Dawley farms (Sprague Dawley animal company) in Madison, Wisconsin in 1925. These albino rats are used extensively in medical research.

12. How are Sprague Dawley rats different from Wistar rats?

Ans: These are less active, calm and easy to handle in comparison to Wistar rats. Wistar rats have wider head, long ears, and the tail length always shorter than that of the body length. Sprague Dawley rats have longer and narrower head, longer tail, which may be equal or longer than the body length (Fig. 1.2).

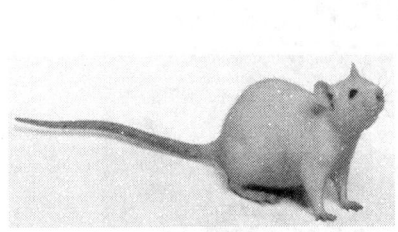
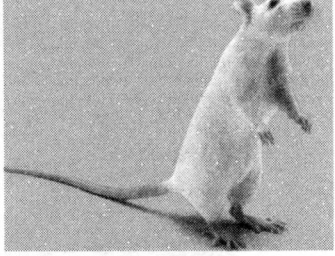

Wistar rat   Sprague Dawley rat

Fig. 1.2: Two most commonly used strains of rat, i.e. Wistar rats and Sprague Dawley rats

13. Which is the most commonly employed strain of mice in pharmacology?

Ans: Swiss albino mice.

14. Why are Swiss albino mice so called?

Ans: These mice are the progeny of two male and seven female albino mice obtained by Dr. Clara Lynch of the Rockefeller Institute from a colleague in Switzerland. Today these are widely used in research. However, erroneously any white mouse is referred to as Swiss, even if it does not originate from true Swiss stock.

15. Describe the main objectives for the selection of animals for various disease models.

Ans: A suitable animal should be selected which follows three main objectives:

    a. Use of an animal phylogenetically (species sharing common ancestors in past) closer to man

    b. Use of an animal with similar anatomy, physiology and biochemistry to that of humans

    c. Use of an animal in which the physiological/ pathophysiological process under investigation is as close as possible to that of man

16. How can sex be determined in rats or mice?

Ans: Sex is most easily determined by anogenital distance. Males normally have a greater distance between the anus and urogenital openings. Male mice also have a larger genital papilla. Scrotum can be easily palpable in males (Fig. 1.3).

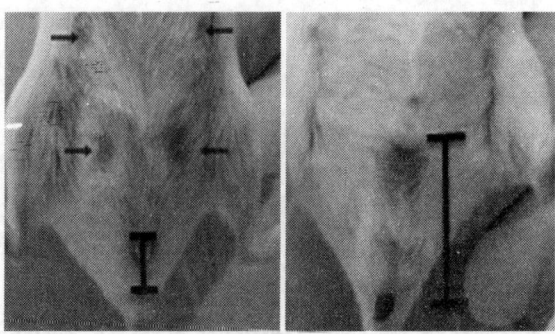

Fig. 1.3: Differentiation of female and male rats

17. **Which animal is selected first for preliminary pharmacological studies?**

Ans: Due to large similarity between mice and human genome (> 90% conserved) and small size, mice are selected first for creating a disease model.

18. **Describe some phenotypic differences between baby rats and mice.**

Ans: There are some phenotypic differences between baby rats and mice:

    a. Baby rats have blunt, broad and large head relative to the body, whereas mice have triangular and smaller head relative to the body

    b. Baby rats have small ears relative to the head, whereas mice have large ears

    c. In baby rats, hind paw and body ratio is larger as compared to mice

    d. Tail is thick and shorter than body length in baby rat, while mice have thin and larger or tail in same length as compared to the body

FOR POSTGRADUATES

19. **Which animal is more suitable for behavioral studies?**

Ans: Rats should be preferred for behavioral studies because of their docility, adaptability to new surroundings, tendency to explore, ease of training, responsiveness to reward punishment and a variety of sensory cues. Mice are not as proficient as rats for running on mazes and are therefore, not used as often. However, mice are also used for behavioral studies.

20. **What are the main characteristics of Guinea pigs?**

Ans: Guinea pigs are docile in nature, more resistant to hypoxia than rat and mice. They are very susceptible to tuberculosis and anaphylactic shock. They are also highly sensitive to histamine. They seem to be closer to man than rats.

21. **In which pharmacological experiments, Guinea pigs are preferred animals?**

Ans: These are preferred animals for the following experiments:

a. For evaluation of bronchodilator compounds and local anesthetics
b. In immunology particularly in hypersensitivity testing
c. These have highly sensitive cochlea, therefore, used for hearing related experiments
d. Being docile in nature and being more resistant to hypoxia than rat and mice, these are suitable for experiment related to oxygen consumption.
e. Suitable host for mycobacterial infection
f. More resemblance to human than rat, so used for study of isoniazid toxicity

22. Why Guinea pigs are preferred animals for inducing pulmonary disease models?

Ans: Guinea pigs respond to histamine with characteristic bronchospasm and asphyxia similar to anaphylactic shock in humans.

23. What is the preferable weight of guinea pig for experimentation?

Ans: The animals between the weight groups of 300 and 400 gm are preferred. The large animals (> 600 gm) are difficult to prepare for surgery. The young animals (< 3 months old, < 250 gm) are in a rapid development phase which increases the variability.

24. Why is it essential to add vitamin C in the chow for Guinea pig (*Cavia porcellus*)?

Ans: Guinea pig is herbivorous and eats green foods, seeds and roots. In laboratory, feed is provided with a ready-made chow diet, and Guinea pigs are not able to synthesize vitamin C (Ascorbic acid), so it is essential to add vitamin C in the chow.

25. What is the main characteristic of rabbit for experimental pharmacology?

Ans: Rabbit is a standard animal for pyrogen testing of all solutions for human medical use. Rabbit is very sensitive to histamine and has the ability to taste water, a characteristic absent in rats. It is the only known animal from which tubules of the kidney can be dissected with intact basement membrane.

26. Which animal has the coronary circulatory and cardiovascular systems very similar to humans?

Ans: Pigs have very similar coronary circulatory system to human beings. The size and shape of pig's cardiovascular system is also very similar to that in humans.

27. Which animal is preferred for cardiovascular studies?

Ans: Pig is the ideal animal for CVS studies because its anatomy is very close to humans. The collateral blood vessels are formed like in humans and are prone to arrhythmias. But the major limitation is the presence of thick fatty layer around the heart.

28. Write the feature of rats for cardiovascular studies.

Ans: Rats do not develop collateral blood vessels; therefore, these are very useful to study the effects of ischemia. These are resistant to arrhythmias and revert to normal sinus rhythm spontaneously.

29. Which are the different mammals that are employed in studying arrhythmia-related studies?

Ans: The mammals are divided into two groups:
   a. **Rat, Guinea pig, rabbit and cat:** These have relatively small heart and capable of restoring ventricular fibrillation to normal rhythm in a spontaneous manner.
   b. **Dogs and monkey:** These have relatively larger hearts and are not inclined to spontaneous defibrillation.

30. Why cold blooded animals like frog are not preferred for studying arrhythmias?

Ans: Arrhythmias in cold blooded animals are very different from those produced in higher animals including humans.

31. For which disease models, rats and mice are not suitable?

Ans: Rodents are not preferred for the following disease models:
   a. **Arrhythmias:** As rodents are normally resistant to development of arrhythmias.
   b. Rodents do not possess the vomiting center, so these are not the good choice for evaluating antiemetic agents.

c. **Atherosclerosis:** Rats are generally resistant to atherogenesis, although lipid containing lesions can be produced in rats with great efforts.

32. What are spontaneously hypertensive rats?

Ans: These are derived from Wistar rats and these show an exaggerated cardiovascular responsiveness to environmental alerting stimuli, i.e. noise, vibration, and light. Due to the exaggerated cardiovascular response, the animals develop spontaneous hypertension in response to external stimuli.

33. What are Dahl salt-sensitive rats?

Ans: These genetically salt sensitive rats were developed by Dahl and his associates. These rats develop hypertension, when exposed to a high-salt diet. The hypertension is maintained even if the salt is withdrawn.

34. What do you understand by knock-in and knock-out mice?

Ans: Knock-out and knock-in mice have been developed for studying the pathophysiological effects of a particular gene in a disease. In knock-out mice, a selective gene is taken out, whereas in knock-in mice, gene of interest is introduced into the mice.

35. Who created the first knock-out mouse?

Ans: The first knock-out mouse was created by Mario R Capecchi, Martin Evans and Oliver Smithies in 1989, for which they were awarded the Nobel Prize for Medicine in 2007.

36. What are BB rats?

Ans: BB stands for Bio-Breeding and is developed by Bio-Breeding laboratories. This breed has a genetic predisposition to develop IDDM and hence, spontaneously develop the symptoms of glycosuria, hyperglycemia and hypoinsulinemia by the age of 3 months.

37. What are NOD mice?

Ans: NOD stands for non-obese diabetic and it also develops spontaneous diabetes similar to that of BB rats. Though inflammatory cells may be seen in the pancreas (insulitis) of all animals, however, over diabetes develops only in 80 % of female and 20 % of male rats. The apparent failure of significant number of NOD mice to develop diabetes and marked sex differences in disease development are the two main differences between NOD mice and BB rats. The inbred NOD mouse is considered to be a good model for type 1 diabetes mellitus.

38. Which are the other animals those develop IDDM spontaneously?

Ans: New Zealand white rabbit has shown incidences of spontaneous diabetes, approximately 18% in some colonies. IDDM also develops in 50% of the breeding colony of Guinea pigs. Diabetes also develops in Chinese hamsters with variable and unpredictable severity.

39. Where are BALB/c mice mainly employed?

Ans: BALB/c mice are mainly useful for research in cancer and immunology. Furthermore, these are very useful for the production of monoclonal antibodies. These display high levels of anxiety and are relatively resistant to diet-induced *atherosclerosis*, making them a useful model for the cardiovascular research.

40. What are athymic nude mice?

Ans: The athymic nude mouse lacks thymus gland, therefore, the immune system is very weak in these animals. Due to this feature, these are commonly used in oncology (cancer) and immunogenetics.

41. What does STR/1N represent?

Ans: STR/1N mouse strain was characterized by Walton. Male mice develop osteoarthritis much earlier and more consistently than the female mice without dietary restriction. Additionally, these also develop obesity.

42. What does New Zealand Black/White F1 (B/W) represent?

Ans: This inbred strain develops nephritis similar to that in human systematic lupus erythematous and shows mononuclear cell infiltration in salivary and lachrymal glands such as in human Sjögren's syndrome.

43. What does New Zealand Black (NZB) mouse represent?

Ans: NZB mouse develops spontaneous autoimmune disease with autoimmune hemolytic anemia, glomerulonephritis, splenomegaly, lymphoproliferative disorder and peptic ulceration.

44. What does Obese strain chicken (OS chicken) represent?

Ans: The OS chicken is the best studied model for an organ specific, spontaneously occurring autoimmune disease, viz. spontaneously occurring autoimmune thyroiditis which closely resembles human hashimoto thyroiditis.

45. What are the characteristic features of New Zealand Black (NZB) mouse?

Ans: NZB mouse develops spontaneous autoimmune disease such as autoimmune hemolytic anemia and splenomegaly.

46. What do MRL/lpr mice represent?

Ans: MRL/lpr mice spontaneously develop a severe disease with many symptoms closely related to human SLE, i.e. hypergammaglobulinemia and glomerulonephritis.

47. What are Fatty Zucker rats?

Ans: Fatty Zucker (fa/fa) rats are mostly used as model of NIDDM due to development of insulin resistance.

48. What are ob/ob mice?

Ans: These mice are the models of obesity diabetes syndrome. The symptoms of these mice include hyperphagia, increased proportion of body fat, hyperinsulinemia and hyperglycemia.

49. Which are the animals of spontaneous NIDDM-like syndrome without developing ketosis?

Ans: Fatty Zucker (fa/fa) rats and ob/ob mice are the models of spontaneous NIDDM-like syndrome without developing ketosis.

50. What does WDF/Ta-fa rat represent?

Ans: WDF/Ta-fa rat, commonly referred to Wistar fatty rat, is a genetically obese, hyperglycemic rat established by transferring the fatty (fa) gene from the Zucker rat to the Wistar Kyoto rat. These rats are more glucose tolerant and insulin resistant than Zucker rats.

51. Which are the animals of spontaneous NIDDM-like syndrome with ketosis?

Ans: db/db mice and Keeshond dog.

52. What does db/db represent?

Ans: These are the models of diabetic mice. The db/db mouse develops a severe diabetic syndrome and significant nephropathy.

53. What does eSS-rat represent?

Ans: The occurrence of spontaneous diabetes in a colony of rats called eSS-rat, was reported by Tarres et al (1981). The animals show tolerance tests from the age of 2 months onwards. Six months old rats show disruption of the pancreatic islet architecture and fibrosis of the stroma.

54. What does SHR/N-cp rat represent?

Ans: SHR/N-cp is a homozygous (cp/cp) rat which exhibits obesity, mild hypertension, hyperinsulinemia, and glucose intolerance.

55. What does BHE rat represent?

Ans: BHE rat is a model in which the diabetic state is manifested only at maturity. BHE rats develop hyperinsulinemia at the 50 days of age. These exhibit hyperinsulinemia with reduced pancreatic insulin stores and also show hyperglycemia and hyperlipidemia.

56. What does KK mouse represent?

Ans: Iwatsuka et al. (1970) reported yellow KK mice (also named KK-A^y mice) carrying the yellow obese gene. These mice develop marked adiposity and diabetic symptoms.

57. What does NZO mouse represent?

Ans: NZO strain was developed by selective inbreeding of obese mice from a mixed colony. NZO mice develop obesity, mild hyperglycemia, glucose intolerance, hyperinsulinemia and insulin resistance.

58. What do BL/6 obese mice represent?

Ans: BL/6 obese mice are characterized by marked obesity, hyperphagia, transient hyperglycemia and markedly elevated plasma insulin concentrations associated with an increase in number and size of beta cells in the islets of Langerhans of pancreas.

59. What are RICO rats?

Ans: RICO rats are the strains of genetically hypercholesrolemic, normotriglyceridemic and non-obese rats. This strain is used to study the effects of hypolipidemic drugs, particularly those that are designed to decrease the plasma concentration of chylomicrons and LDL.

60. What are WHHL rabbit?

Ans: Watanabe et al described a strain of rabbit with hereditary hyperlipidemia. These are used to study the development of atherosclerosis as well as the histological and functional changes of the aorta.

61. What does DBA/2FG-pcy mouse represent?

Ans: DBA/2FG-pcy mouse develops numerous cysts in kidney cortex and medulla, a progressive anemia and an elevation of blood urea nitrogen. These have been useful as spontaneous model of progressive renal failure.

62. What does senescence-accelerated mouse (SAM) represent?

Ans: SAM strain is recommended to study age-dependent memory deficits.

63. What does TGR (mREN2) 27 rat represent?

Ans: TGR (mREN2) 27 is a transgenic rat with elevated renin angiotensin system and used as a monogenetic model in hypertension.

64. What does TGR (ASrAOGEN) 680 represent?

Ans: TGR (ASrAOGEN) 680 is a transgenic rat line with specific down regulation of astroglial synthesis of angiotensinogen and exhibits decreased brain angiotensinogen. It represents the centrally inactivated angiotensin system.

65. What does NC/NgaTnd mouse represent?

Ans: NC/NgaTnd mouse is an inbred strain originated from Japanese fancy mice. These develop itchy dermatitis spontaneously in an air-unregulated conventional circumstance at 6 to 8 weeks of age. It is used as a good model for atopic dermatitis.

66. What does asebia (ab/ab) mouse represent?

Ans: The asebia (ab/ab) mouse was first described by Gates and Kasarek (1965). It is characterized by defective sebaceous glands and other cutaneous abnormalities. It is a good model for scarring and alopecia.

67. What does chakragati (ckr) mouse represent?

Ans: Chakragati mouse (ckr) is a transgenic insertional mutant, which displays lateral circling and locomotor hyperactivity. It is used to study the aspects of neuropsychiatric disorders associated with dopaminergic abnormalities.

68. What do transgenic Cu/Zn-SOD mice represent?

Ans: Transgenic Cu/Zn-SOD mice overexpress the gene encoding copper/zinc superoxide dismutase, which is also overexpressed in human Down syndrome.

69. What does TSK mouse represent?

Ans: Tight skin (TSK) is an autosomal dominant mutation located on mouse chromosome 2 and is associated with an intragenic duplication of the fibrillin 1 (Fbn 1) gene. Mutant mice (TSK/+) display tightness of skin in the interscapular region, lung emphysema, myocardial hypertrophy, skeletal overgrowth, and kyphosis.
   a. The tight skin (TSK) mouse is a genetic model of pulmonary emphysema associated with right ventricular hypertrophy.
   b. It has been used as a model for various human diseases associated with abnormalities of the connective tissue.

70. What are the characteristic features of New Zealand Black/ White (B/W) F1 mouse?

Ans: These animals develop nephrites similar to that of human systemic lupus erythematous (SLE). Furthermore, in these animals, the inflammation is present in salivary and lacrimal gland similar to Sjögren's syndrome.

71. Which is the suitable laboratory animal for evaluating antiemetic activity?

Ans: Dog is the only suitable species to test antiemetic drugs. Rodents cannot be used because these lack vomiting center.

72. What is the hematological data of commonly used laboratory animals?

Ans:

Hematological data			
Parameters	Mouse	Rat	Rabbit
RBC ($\times 10$ V/mm^3)	7–12.5	7–10	4–7
Hb (gm/dl)	10.2–16.6	11–18	10–15.5
WBC ($\times 10^3$/mm^3)	6–15	6–17	9–11
Neutrophils (%)	10–40	9–34	20–75
Platelets ($\times 10^3$/mm^3)	160–410	500–1300	250–656
Biochemical data			
Protein (gm/dl)	3.5–7.2	5.6–7.6	5.4–7.5
Albumin (gm/dl)	2.5–4.8	2.8–4.8	2.7–4.6
Glucose (mg/dl)	62–175	50–135	75–150
Urea nitrogen (mg/dl)	12–28	15–21	17–23.5
Creatine (mg/dl)	0.3–1	0.2–0.8	0.8–1.8
Cholesterol (mg/dl)	26–82	40–130	35–53

2

General Animal Behavior and their Significance in Experimental Pharmacology

FOR UNDERGRADUATES AND POSTGRADUATES

1. Define catalepsy and catatonia.

Ans: Both catatonia and catalepsy represent intense rigidity in the body. Catalepsy is the abnormal maintenance of distorted posture, often called 'waxy flexibility'. The time it takes to return to normal posture gives an indication of extent of catalepsy. Catalepsy is generally a symptom of certain nervous disorders such as Parkinson's disease, epilepsy and or conditions like cocaine withdrawal. Catalepsy is generally used to describe abnormal position in humans.

On the other hand, catatonia describes the inability to correct its abnormal posture in rodents over a prolonged period of time (Fig. 2.1). The drugs that block dopaminergic system in the nigrostriatal pathway in the brain produce catalepsy.

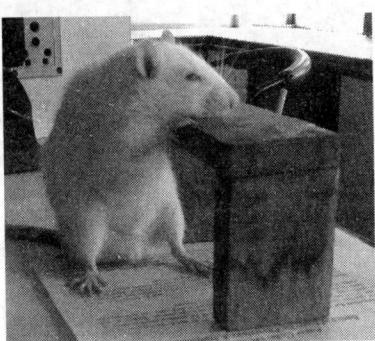

Fig. 2.1: Demonstration of catatonia in rat on chlorpromazine administration

2. **What is the utility of catatonia in experimental pharmacology?**

Ans: Catalepsy is of interest to the researchers because of its similarity to symptoms of human disorders such as Parkinsonism, catatonic schizophrenia and brain damage involving parts of the basal ganglia. In addition, catalepsy is one of the behavioral tools mostly used by neuroscientists to study the behavioral mechanisms of neurochemical systems.

3. **Write the practical application of catatonia development in drug evaluation in experimental pharmacology.**

Ans: Experimentally, the drugs blocking dopaminergic pathway (antipsychotic, e.g. chlorpromazine) are administered to induce catatonia in rats. The anticholinergic drugs (atropine) prevent chlorpromazine induce catatonia in rats.

4. **What do you understand by righting reflex?**

Ans: It is the reflex phenomenon in which rodents regain their posture, when placed on dorsal surface (means on back) (Fig. 2.2).

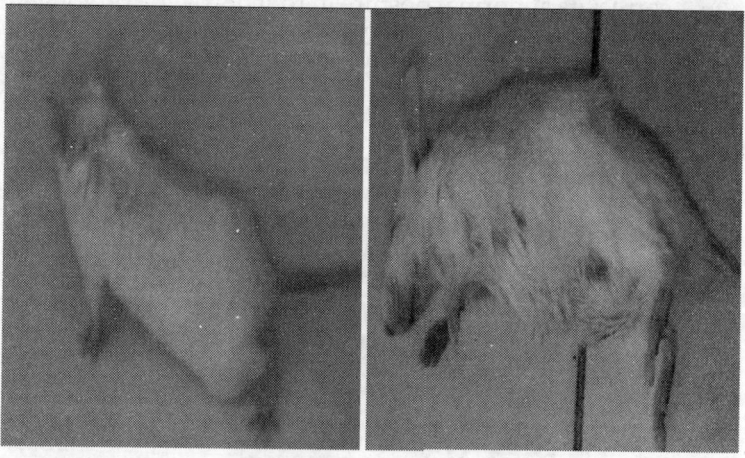

Fig. 2.2: Demonstration of loss of righting reflex on administration of sedative

5. **What is the significance of righting reflex?**

Ans: Righting reflex is a simple test and is widely used to screen the compounds with sedative properties. To assess the righting reflex, the mouse is normally placed on its back on a flat surface or V-shaped enclosure. The time taken to regain right posture itself (up to a maximum of 30 seconds) is measured.

6. **What do you understand by loss of righting reflex and what is its significance?**

Ans: The *"loss of righting reflex"* is the term mainly used to denote the sleep of an animal. When animal is placed on its back, it immediately recovers from that position. However, during loss of righting reflex, it fails to recover. The proper posture, when placed its back. It is defined as the loss of postural reaction in which the animal cannot correct its posture, when kept on its back.

7. **What is Straub's tail? Write its significance.**

Ans: A severe spasm of the anal sphincter (sacrococcygeus muscle) resulting in erection of the tail (about 90°) is termed Straub's tail (Fig. 2.3). It is generally an indication of intense CNS stimulation.

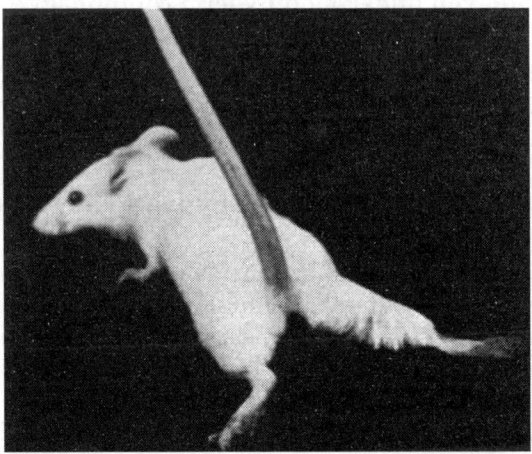

Fig. 2.3: Demonstration of Straub's tail on administration of PTZ in mice

8. **Write the significance of Straub's tail.**

Ans: a. This phenomenon is observed during pentylenetetrazole (PTZ)-induced convulsions. The antiepileptic drugs prevent PTZ-induced Struab's tail and convulsions.

b. Furthermore, intracerebroventricular injection of morphine in animals also produces erection of tail. This effect is mediated via activation of supraspinal µ-opioid receptors and is inhibited by supraspinal kappa-opioid receptors. This test was formerly employed to detect morphine in biological fluids.

9. **What do you understand by spontaneous motor activity?**

Ans: Motor activity is a good parameter for studying the effects of pharmacological agents on central nervous system. Spontaneous motor activity includes different types of movements such as locomotion, rearing (raise itself upright on its hind legs), sniffing (to use the sense via smelling, as in savoring or investigating), grooming (to remove dirt and parasites from the skin, fur, or feathers of another animal), eating and drinking.

FOR POSTGRADUATES

10. **What do you understand by term coprophagy?**

Ans: It is defined as ingestion of feces by the animal including eating feces of other species (hetero-specifics), of other individuals of same species (allo-coprophagy), or its own (auto-coprophagy).

11. **What is the significance of coprophagy in experimental pharmacology?**

Ans: Because rodents exhibit the phenomenon of coprophagy, therefore, the animals cannot be kept in a fasting state just by placing an animal in a cage without giving the food. The rodents tend to consume their fecal matter and hence, utilize the undigested food in fecal matter. Therefore, that state cannot be called a true fasting state.

12. How can be rodents kept in a fasting state?

Ans: The rodents must be fasted by placing them in a specially designed metabolic cage (Fig. 2.4) in which fecal matter passes down and collects in a separate container. Therefore, animals are unable to consume the undigested food present in fecal matter in the form of coprophagy.

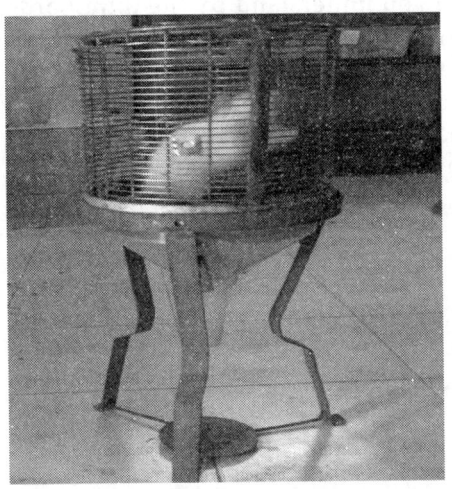

Fig. 2.4: Metabolic cage for keeping the rodents in fasting state

13. Name the experiments in which animals must be in fasting state.

Ans: The animals must be in fasting state for the following experiments:

   a. Diabetes mellitus related experiments in which fasting glucose levels are measured in blood/plasma.
   b. Before inducing ulcerative colitis or inflammatory bowel disease
   c. For plotting the DRC of agonist using fundus preparation

14. What do you understand by the term cannibalism?

Ans: Cannibalism is defined as the act of killing and eating its own species. The rodents generally exhibit the phenomenon of cannibalism.

15. What is the significance of cannibalism in experimental pharmacology?

Ans: Cannibalism phenomenon is shown under different conditions and for different reasons. Cannibalism represents the hunger behavior and neurological disorder (disturbances like stress and depression).

16. What do you understand by the term Lordosis?

Ans: Lordosis is defined as female mating posture in oestrus, a reflexive behavior that is triggered by a touch on the lower back, flanks or genital region. Vulva which normally faces the floor, rotates almost 90° to the vertical, i.e. to backward facing position (Fig. 2.5).

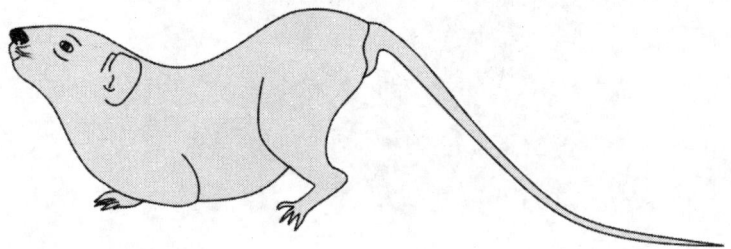

Fig. 2.5: Demonstration of female Lordosis behavior

17. What do you understand by the term Lordosis avoiding behavior?

Ans: Lordosis avoidance behavior is an avoidance of reflexive behavior that is triggered by a touch on the lower back, flanks, or genital region. Loss of the Lordosis can be the result of stress, depression, hormonal imbalance, trauma, degenerative processes, congenital defects, posture or post-surgical complications.

18. What is the significance of Lordosis in experimental pharmacology?

Ans: Lordosis behavior is used for evaluation of different drugs in neuronal disorders including stress, depression, trauma, degenerative processes, congenital defects, posture or post-surgical complications.

19. What do you mean by classical conditioning?

Ans: Classical conditioning is the procedure in which an initially neutral stimulus (e.g. bell or alarm as conditional stimulus) is repeatedly paired with an unconditional stimulus (e.g. food) and a response is noted (e.g. salivation). The result of pairing conditioned stimulus with unconditioned stimulus during trial (training) period is that the conditional stimulus (bell alone) in the absence of unconditioned stimulus (food) begins to elicit a conditioned response (salivation) during test period.

20. Write the significance of classical conditioning.

Ans: Classical conditioning is an important behavioral phenomenon and is used to study learning and memory. It is also used to study other neurodisturbances including stress, anxiety and depression.

21. What do you mean by conditioned reflex?

Ans: Conditioned reflex is the other name for a conditional response, i.e. the response that is elicited by a neutral, conditional stimulus (in the absence of unconditioned stimulus) after classical conditioning has taken place. The term "reflex" is used here to connect the concept with the tradition of studying reflexes in physiology.

22. What do you mean by fear potentiated startle response?

Ans: Fear potentiated startle is an exaggerated startle (shock like, freezing) reaction to a sudden stimulus provided to an already stressed animal. The startle response is a defensive reflex evoked by unexpected and intense stimuli (for instance, a loud noise). For example, application of sound of very high intensity to anxious animals triggers a state of panic, which is manifested in the form of fear potentiated startle response.

23. What do you mean by learned helplessness?

Ans: Learned helplessness occurs when an animal is subjected to an aversive stimulus from which it cannot escape. Eventually, the animal stops trying to avoid the stimulus and behaves as if it is utterly helpless to change the situation. Even when the opportunities to escape are presented, the learned helplessness prevents the escape actions of animal.

24. **What is the significance of learned helplessness in experimental pharmacology?**

Ans: The theory of learned helplessness is applied to many conditions and behaviors including depression. In laboratory, the development of learned helplessness has been associated with development of depression. The drugs that prevent learned helplessness prevent the development of depression.

25. **What do you mean by reinforcement?**

Ans: Reinforcement is a stimulus which is added in a typical conditioning procedure and it increases or decreases the frequency of subsequent responses. The reinforcement may be a reward or a punishment. For example, pressing a lever in chamber delivers food from food dispenser and induces positive reinforcement. On the other hand, pressing a lever in chamber delivers footshock and induces negative reinforcement.

26. **What do you mean by negative reinforcement?**

Ans: Negative reinforcement is a type of punishment and its withdrawal from the environment immediately increases the response. In other words, withdrawal of this stimulus serves to strengthen the response.

27. **What do you mean by positive reinforcement?**

Ans: Positive reinforcement is a reward and its addition in the environment immediately increases the desired response. In other words, administration of this stimulus serves to strengthen the response and increases the likelihood of its occurrence again.

28. **What do you mean by passive avoidance and what is its significance?**

Ans: In this test, animals learn to avoid an environment in which an aversive stimulus (such as a footshock) was previously delivered. This is a fear-aggravated test and is used to evaluate learning and memory in rodents. In this test, animal is given a shock in a chamber and animal fears this chamber, therefore, avoids entering the chamber. It is a type of fear learning in which animal remembers the past experience in the chamber. However, in memory disorders, animal fails to remember the shock and there is no avoidance for entering the chamber.

29. What do you understand by thigmotaxis?

Ans: It was described by Barnett (1963). Thigmotaxis is a special phenomenon which means that rats have a tendency to remain close to the walls of the cages. The degree of thigmotaxis is usually considered as an index of anxiety in mice.

On the other hand, the non-anxious rats tend to move in centre of chamber and do not show thigmotaxis.

30. What is hole board test?

Ans: Hole board test generally assesses the exploratory behavior of the animals and is a useful method for screening the potential anxiolytic drugs. The test is based on the assumption that head-dipping activity (exploratory activity) of the animals is inversely proportional to their anxiety state.

The non-anxious rats tend to explore the board and peep through the holes of chamber. Therefore, higher number of head dips (peeping through holes) indicates exploratory behavior and non-anxious state (Fig. 2.6).

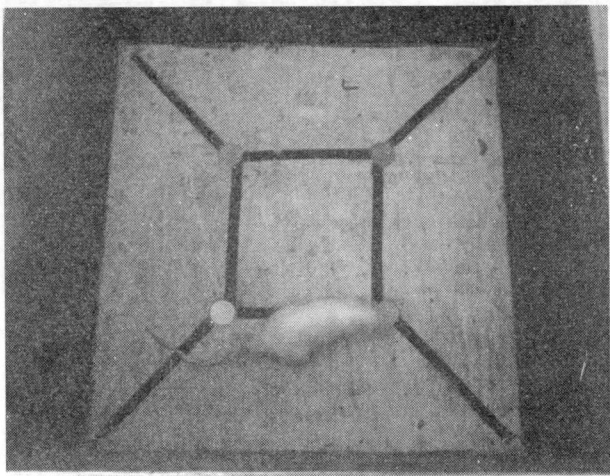

Fig. 2.6: Demonstration of exploratory behavior of non-anxious rat in terms of head dips in hole made on the floor of hole board apparatus

31. What is open field test?

Ans: Open field test simultaneously measures locomotion, exploration and anxiety. The non-anxious mice tend to explore the board and have increased number of line crossings and more number of rearings. Furthermore, there is increased number of central square entries and the duration of time spent in the central square as compared to peripheral area in non-anxious mice (Fig. 2.7).

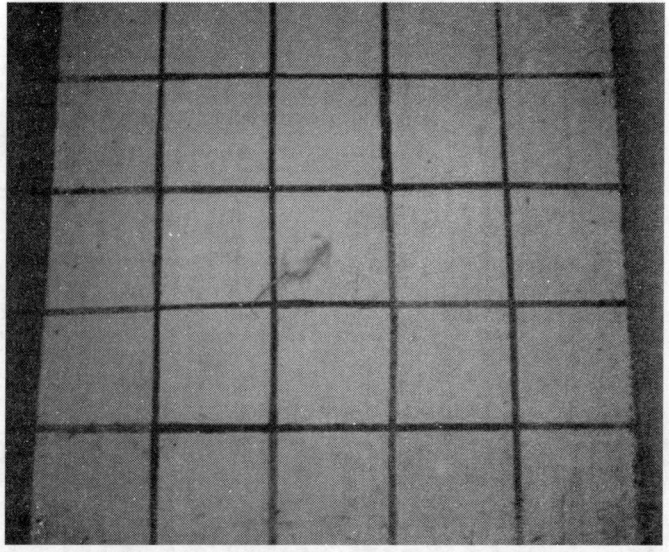

Fig. 2.7: Demonstration of non-anxious mouse in open field board as the animal is staying more in the central squares as compared to peripheral area

General Pharmacological Techniques

3

1. **What are the gastrointestinal routes of administration of drugs?**

Ans: a. Oral (per os)—through the mouth (Fig. 3.1)
b. Gavage—into the stomach via a tube or gavage needle
c. Rectal (per rectum)—into the rectum via the anus

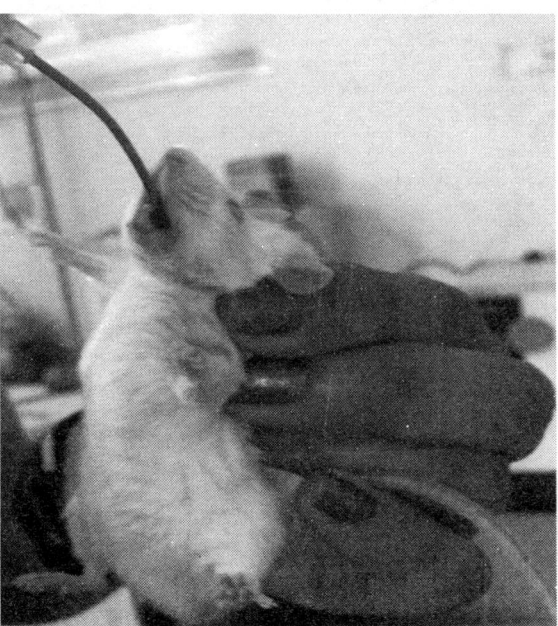

Fig. 3.1: Administration of drug in mouse by oral route

2. **What is the most common route of administration in rodents?**

Ans: Intraperitoneal route is the most commonly employed route for administering drugs in animals.

3. **What are the characteristics of intraperitoneal (IP) route?**

Ans: In this route, the drug is deposited in the peritoneal cavity from which the drug is absorbed into the blood capillaries. The peritoneal cavity is richly supplied by blood capillaries which results in rapid absorption of injected drug.

4. **What is the procedure of IP administration?**

Ans: The needle is inserted into lower abdomen on either side of the midline just above the right or left leg. Once through the skin, the needle is raised to a 45° angle and allowed to penetrate the muscle wall of peritoneal cavity through about 1 cm (Fig. 3.2).

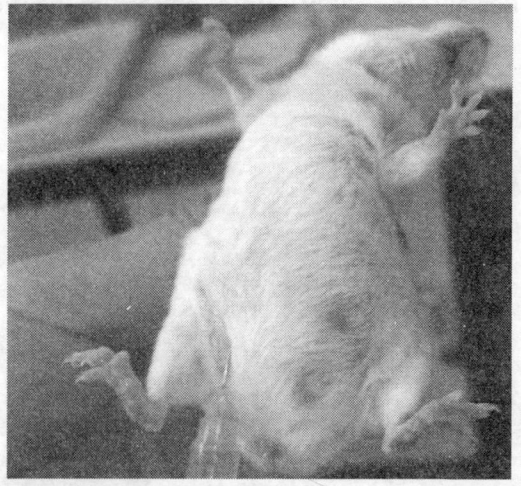

Fig. 3.2: Administration of drug in mouse by intraperitoneal route

5. **How is it ensured that the drug has not actually gone to gastrointestinal tract during IP administration?**

Ans: During IP administration, there is possibility that needle punctures the blood vessels or intestine. Therefore, when the needle is placed correctly, the syringe should be pulled back slightly. The presence of blood or abdominal content indicates the wrong position of needle and therefore drug should not be administered.

6. **What is the limitation of this route?**

Ans: In this route, a certain amount of variability is introduced due to difference in drug absorption depending upon where the drug is deposited in the peritoneum. Other limitations include the sensitivity of peritoneal tissue to irritating substances and less tolerance to solutions of non-physiological pH.

7. **Is this route also a favorable route of administering drugs in humans?**

Ans: Intraperitoneal route is rarely used in humans because of danger of intraperitoneal infection.

8. **What are the characteristics of intramuscular route of administration?**

Ans: There is slow and even absorption over a period of time when drugs are injected by intramuscular route. The drugs are absorbed within 10–30 minutes of injection. In rats, < 0.2 ml/site may be injected into the quadriceps or the gluteal muscles. If injection is made into the gluteal muscle, it must be ensured that sciatic nerve is not punctured, which runs along the caudal aspect of the femur (Fig. 3.3).

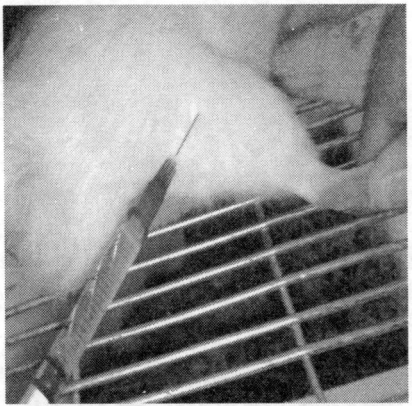

Fig. 3.3: Administration of drug in mouse by intramuscular route in gluteal muscle

9. **Why is intramuscular route not recommended in mice?**

Ans: Intramuscular route not recommended in mice due to their small muscle mass.

10. **How many veins are present in the rat/mice tail?**

Ans: There are four veins present in tail:

a. Two dorsal tail veins—on the dorsal surface
b. Two ventral tail veins—on the sides of tail

11. **What are the characteristics and advantages of intravenous (i.v.) route over other routes?**

Ans: In this route, the drug is administered directly into the venous bloodstream by injecting in the tail veins of mouse (Fig. 3.4). Solutions of high/low pH or irritating substance can be administered intravenously provided that the rate of injection is kept slow and precautions are taken to avoid spillage of the solution outside the vein. Furthermore, isotonic solutions of quite large volume can be administered by this route.

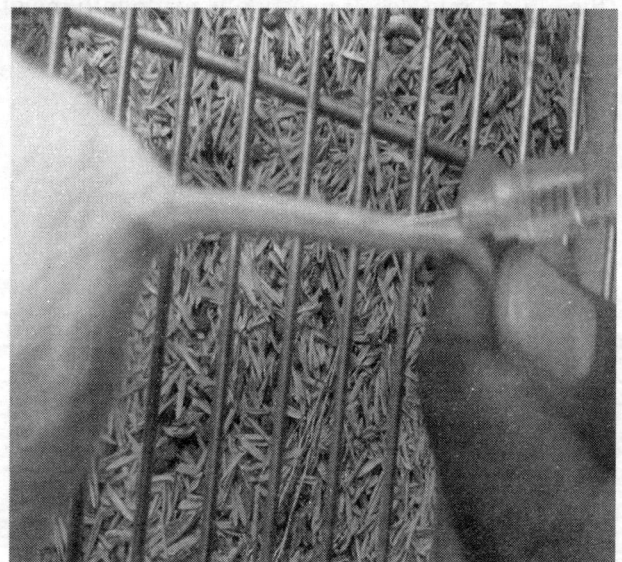

Fig. 3.4: Administration of drug in tail vein by intravenous route

12. What are side effects of intravenous administration in rats?

Ans: If solutions are administrated intravenously, hemodynamic changes and pulmonary oedema may occur. A very rapid injection can produce cardiovascular failure and may be lethal. Furthermore, only isotonic solutions may be administered by this route.

13. What is the size of needle used for intravenous administration in experimental studies?

Ans: Generally, the principle of selection of needle size (length and bore) is based upon the size of the vein, i.e. the bore size selected should have lesser diameter than the vein. In the experimental studies, needles between 10 and 50 mm in length and 17 and 27 G bore are preferred.

14. What do you mean by subcutaneous route of drug administration?

Ans: Subcutaneous administrations are made into the loose skin over the interscapular or inguinal area. Anesthesia is generally not required (Fig. 3.5).

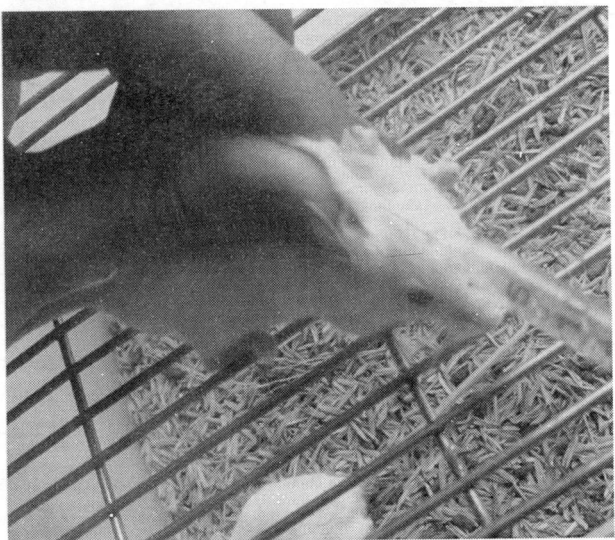

Fig. 3.5: Subcutaneous administration of drug in interscapular region in mouse

15. What are the different needles used for different route of administration?

Ans: The following table provides the basic information on injection techniques, needle size, and recommended injection volumes for common laboratory animals.

Species	Oral	Intravenous	Intraperitoneal	Intramuscular	Subcutaneous
Mouse	20 ml/kg < 22 G	10 ml/kg < 25 G	20 ml/kg < 23 G	Generally not recommended Quadriceps/ posterior thigh: 0.05 ml total; 25 G	20 ml/kg < 25 G
Rat	20 ml/kg < 23 G	5 ml/kg < 23 G	10 ml/kg < 21 G	Generally not recommended Quadriceps/ posterior thigh: 0.1 ml total; ~23–25 G	5 ml/kg < 20 G
Rabbit	10 ml/kg by gavage < 21 G	2 ml/kg < 20 G	4 ml/kg < 20 G	Quadriceps/ posterior thigh: 0.05 ml total; 25 G	1 ml/kg < 20 G

Hull RM (1995). Human and Experimental Toxicology 14, 305–307.

16. What is the common method for collecting blood from rodents?

Ans: A common method to collect blood (0.1 ml) from rats and mice is to remove the tip of tail for repeated sampling; the blood clot has to be removed to get fresh capillary blood.

17. When does retro-orbital bleeding method is employed?

Ans: It is generally employed to collect the blood in tail-less animals, e.g. Hamster. However, it may also be employed to collect large volume of blood from rats and mice.

18. How blood collection can be done from retro-orbital sinus?

Ans: The rodent is anesthetized, and then manually restrained on a solid surface by holding it gently, but firmly by the nape of the neck. By pressing down with the thumb and forefinger in the occipital area and pulling back the skin, a capillary tube/pipette is pushed with a rotating movement through the conjunctiva medially, laterally or dorsally. Blood is allowed to flow by capillary action into the capillary tube/pipette (Fig. 3.6).

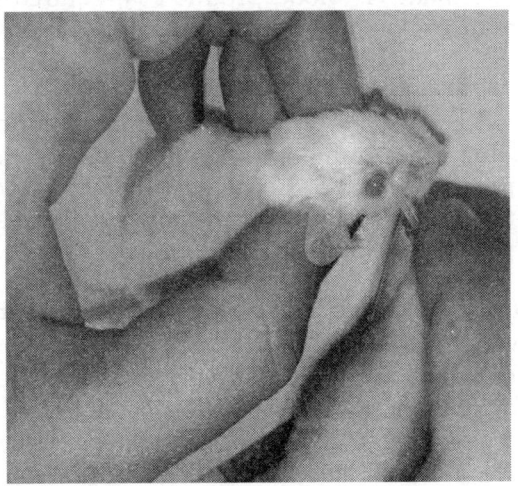

Fig. 3.6: Blood withdrawal technique from retro-orbital sinus plexus

19. **What are the limitations of blood withdrawal techniques from retro-obital sinus?**

Ans: Several side effects such as retro-orbital haemotoma with subsequent pressure on the eye cannot be completely excluded. This pressure can damage the optic nerve.

20. **What is the upper limit of blood volume that may be withdrawn from animals?**

Ans: The total blood volume is 6 to 7% of total body weight (2 ml in mice and 18–20 ml in rats). Not more than 10% of total blood volume (0.2 ml in mice and 2 ml in rats) should be removed within 24 hours period.

21. **What are the repeated blood withdrawal limits with larger blood volume required?**

Ans: Not more than 10% of the total body volume should be removed after a single puncture. For example, this would equate to removal of 0.2 ml from a 25 gm mouse or 2.0 ml from a 250 gm rat. Removal of larger volumes necessitates longer recovery periods for the animal, or may cause distress or death. More than 10–20% total blood volume may be taken once every 2 weeks. If there is a scientific necessity for removal of more than 1% of the body weight within a two week period, then possible replacement via blood products is required (e.g. fluid administration, red blood cell administration).

22. How is plasma separated from blood?

Ans: Blood is collected in a tube containing anticoagulant. Plasma is separated by spinning a blood sample in a centrifuge (5000 RPM), wherein heavier blood cells settle at the bottom, and blood plasma is collected from the upper layer using a pipette.

23. What is the difference between plasma and serum?

Ans: Plasma is the liquid part of blood, in which blood cells, nutrients and hormones are present. Serum is the fluid part of blood, which does not contain the clotting factors and blood cells. The major difference between plasma and serum is absence of fibrinogen in serum.

	Plasma	Serum
1.	Water	Water
2.	Albumin	Albumin
3.	Amino acids	Amino acids
4.	Hormones and enzymes	Hormones and enzymes
5.	Nitrogenous waste	Nitrogenous waste
6.	Nutrients	Nutrients
7.	Gases	Gases
8.	Fibrinogen	–
9.	No cells	No cells

24. How is serum isolated from blood?

Ans: The blood sample in a glass tube is allowed to clot for 1 hour at 37 °C and then kept at 4 °C overnight to allow the clot to contract. Thereafter, the complex is centrifuged at 4000 rpm for 20 minutes at 4 °C to separate serum. It is important that red cells do not lyse as hemolysed products cannot be separated from the serum.

25. What is the significance of plasma separation in biochemical analysis?

Ans: Plasma offers a number of advantages over blood that include:

a. Plasma has longer shelf life than the blood.

b. Frozen plasma can be stored for up to a year.

c. It is more accurate to measure various biochemicals in the plasma than in blood (see biochemical technique chapter).

26. What is the advantage of serum over plasma/blood in biochemical analysis?

Ans: An anticoagulant is added in plasma in order to prevent blood clotting. Presence of anticoagulants in plasma or blood may interfere with the chemical reactions during biochemical analyses. Furthermore, the anticoagulants may draw water out of cells leading to dilution of the sample and change the test results. However, the serum employed for biochemical analyses does not contain anticoagulant and hence, offers advantage over plasma/ blood.

27. What is the storage temperature of blood samples?

Ans: Samples should be frozen immediately at $-70\ °C$ ($-20\ °C$ is not sufficient), if samples are to be stored for a long period.

28. What is the color of plasma? What does red coloration of plasma indicate?

Ans: Plasma is straw or light yellow colored clear liquid and red coloration of plasma indicates hemolysis/rupturing of the RBCs. Hemolysis may be either due to improper handling of the blood sample; or infection or disease in the individual.

29. How can hemolysis be avoided?

Ans: Hemolysis may be avoided by taking the following precautions:

a. By avoiding the sample exposure to extreme heat or cold
b. By allowing the blood to clot completely prior to centrifugation
c. By avoiding vigorous mixing or shaking of tubes
d. By avoiding centrifugation of samples at higher speed or for longer periods

FOR POSTGRADUATES

30. What do you mean by intracranial administration?

Ans: In laboratory experiments, a stereotaxic apparatus and micro-syringe or cannula are employed to facilitate precise drug injection into specific areas of brain tissues. The administration may be either via bolus or continuous administration. The injection may be made:
a. via a surgically implanted cerebral cannula
b. via direct injection
c. via osmotic pump catheter

31. What is intrathecal route of administration?

Ans: In this route, drug is directly injected into the subarachnoid space by administering the drug at the level of spinal cord.

32. What are the different methods to administer the drugs by intrathecal route?

Ans: The drug may be administered by two ways:
a. Surgical method in which drug is administered into the subarachnoid space via chronic intrathecal catheter. But, it is a surgical technique.
b. Direct transcutaneous intrathecal injection in which injection is made between dorsal aspects of L5 and L6, perpendicular to the vertebral column (Fig. 3.7). This site is preferred because injection is restricted to the region, where spinal cord ends and cauda equina begins in order to reduce the possibility of spinal damage.

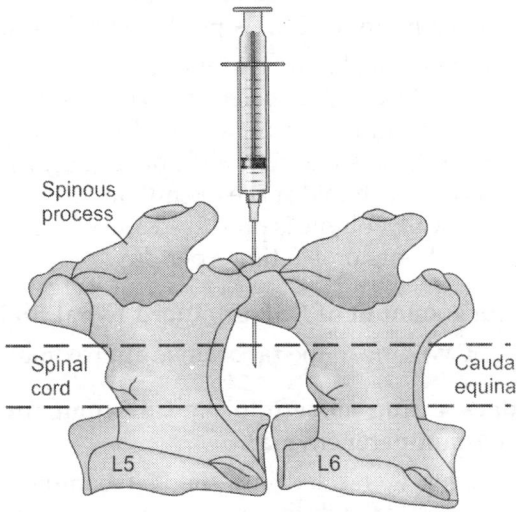

Spinous
process

Spinal
cord

Cauda
equina

L5   L6

Fig. 3.7: Intrathecal administration of drug in rat by direct transcutaneous
injection

**33. How is it verified that needle has entered to subarachnoid
space?**

Ans: When needle enters to the subarachnoid space, a sudden
lateral movement of tail is observed. This reflex is used
as an indicator of successful injection.

**34. What is the importance of intrathecal route of
administration in preclinical studies?**

Ans: In preclinical studies, intrathecal route is used to
distinguish the effect of drugs acting at spinal and
supraspinal levels from extraspinal structures. Furthermore, to study the direct effects of CNS drug on the
spinal cord, it is necessary to apply the drugs at the site
of interest, i.e. at the spinal cord.

**35. What do you mean by intracerebroventricular (ICV)
administration?**

Ans: Administration of drug into cerebrospinal fluid-filled
ventricles (chambers) is called ICV injection.

36. How much amount of CSF is produced by human brain?

Ans: The human brain has no lymphatic system, but produces over a half litre of CSF each day. There is about 140 ml of CSF in the human brain, which fills the four ventricles (20 ml), spinal subarachnoid space (30 ml), and the cranial sub-arachnoid space (90 ml). In the human brain, the entire CSF volume is produced and excreted to blood every 4–5 hours or 4–5 times per day.

37. How much amount of CSF produced by rat brain?

Ans: The CSF volume in the rat brain is approximately 90 µL.

38. How does a drug move into the CSF compartment and into the brain parenchyma?

Ans: When drug is injected into the CSF compartment, the drug passes through these spaces relatively rapidly via convection and bulk flow through the CSF flow tracts. The entry of drug into brain parenchyma from the CSF compartment is mediated by diffusion, a process that is much slower than CSF convection and bulk flow. Moreover, diffusion decreases exponentially with the distance and there is minimal penetration into brain parenchyma, if the distance is more than 1–2 mm from the ependymal surface (ventricle) of brain.

39. What amount of drug should be administered while injecting into CSF?

Ans: Drug concentration in brain parenchyma decreases logarithmically as the distance from the CSF surface is increased. Therefore, if it is required to administer the drug into deep region of brain parenchyma, it is necessary to administer high concentrations of drug into the CSF compartment.

40. How does drug administered through ICV route exit?

Ans: Following the ICV injection of drug, it moves through the CSF flow tracks, and thereafter, it is absorbed into the peripheral bloodstream across the arachnoid villi to enter the general circulation.

41. What do you mean by intracisternal administration?

Ans: It is a type of intracerebroventricular administration in which a drug is administered within one of the subarachnoid cisternae. It usually refers to the introduction of a cannula into the cerebellomedullar cisterna for aspiration of cerebrospinal fluid or injection of drug in the ventricles of the brain. It could be performed by direct injection into the cisterna magna or via a permanently positioned tube.

42. Which blood vessels should be cannulated in Guinea pig for carrying pulmonary experiments?

Ans: For general studies of airway reactivity, jugular vein, femoral vein or inferior vena cava may be cannulated. There is a little importance of type of blood vessels. However, for assessing reflex control of airway reactivity, the blood flow to the brain should not be interrupted. Therefore, the jugular and carotid vessels should not be cannulated.

43. What is the maximum amount of blood that may be withdrawn at a given time?

Ans: A single withdrawal of up to 10% of total blood volume, i.e. 0.2 ml in 25 gm mice (0.008 ml/gm) is generally advocated. If the withdrawal is 20% (0.4 ml), then it may decrease the cardiac output and blood pressure. Withdrawal of blood up to 40% (0.8 ml) induces shock and loss of blood more than 40% may cause mortality. Furthermore, a single withdrawal of up to 15% of total blood volume may be repeated after 3–4 weeks from normal animals.

44. What is the volume of blood that may be withdrawn for repeated sampling?

Ans: Multiple withdrawals of blood samples should not exceed 1% (0.02 ml in 25 gm mice; 0.2 ml in 250 gm rat) of total blood volume (2 ml in mice and 20 ml in rat) in every 24 hours. More frequent withdrawal may produce anemia.

45. How blood collection can be done from tail vein puncture?

Ans: This method is recommended for collecting a large volume of blood sample (up to 2 ml/withdrawal). If the vein is not visible, the tail is dipped into warm water (40 °C). A 23G needle is inserted into the blood vessel and blood is collected using a capillary tube or a syringe with a needle. Silver nitrate ointment/solution is applied to stop the bleeding.

46. What are the precautions to be taken while performing tail vein puncture?

Ans: An attempt should not be made to increase the blood flow by rubbing the tail from the base to the tip. It may result in leukocytosis (increased white blood cell count). Furthermore, restrainer should be washed frequently to avoid/prevent pheromonally-induced stress or cross infection.

47. What do you understand by cardiac puncture technique of blood withdrawal?

Ans: Cardiac puncture represents an accepted method of blood collection from Guinea pigs, gebrils and hamster, when more blood volume required. Animals must be anesthetized and restrained in dorsal position. The needle is inserted under the xyphoid cartilage slightly to the left of midline. The needle is advanced at 20 to 30 degree angle from the horizontal axis to the sternum to enter the heart. The blood is aspirated lightly while advancing. Blood should be withdrawn slowly and the amount must be limited (up to 4 ml in an adult rat), unless euthanasia is planned.

48. What are the different types of plasma collecting tubes?

Ans:

Lavender	Treated with EDTA
Blue	Treated with citrate
Green	Treated with heparin
Grey/yellow	Treated with potassium oxalate/sodium fluoride (not evaluated)

49. What are different types of serum collecting tubes?

Ans:

Red	No anticoagulant
Red with black	Treated with gel that helps to separate the clot

50. What is the maximum withdrawal amount of sample blood volume in rat or mouse?

Ans: **Tail Vein (25–27G):** 50 μl–0.2 ml (mouse); 0.1–2 ml (rat) **Retro-orbital sinus (glass capillary tube):** 0.2 ml with recovery and 0.5 ml without recovery (mouse); up to 2 ml with recovery and 4–10 ml without recovery (rat).

51. Name the commonly employed anesthetics in experimental pharmacology with their doses.

Ans:

Drug (mg/kg)	Mouse	Rat
Ketamine	22–24 i.m.	22–24
Pentobarbitone sodium	35 i.v.; 50 i.p.	25 i.v.; 50 i.p.
Thiopentone sodium	25 i.v.; 50 i.p.	20 i.v.; 24 i.p.
Urethane	–	0.75 i.p.
Chloral hydrate	300–400 mg/kg i.p.	370–450 mg/kg i.p.

52. How is anesthesia checked before conducting surgery?

Ans: The degree of anesthesia is checked by noting loss of reflexes including loss of righting reflex, corneal reflex, digital reflex in a sequential manner.

53. How is the depth of anesthesia monitored by noting the reflexes?

Ans: There is loss of various reflexes as the degree of anesthesia increases in animals in the following order:

  a. *Palpebral reflex*: Touching the eyelids causes blinking.

  b. *Corneal reflex*: Touching the cornea of the eye with a tuft of cotton results in a blink.

  c. *Toe pinch reflex*: Pinching the toe or foot web is followed by withdrawal of the toe due to sensation of pain.

54. What are the other changes introduced as a result of anesthesia?

Ans: The following changes are introduced due to anesthesia:

a. *Muscle tone* decreases as the depth of anesthesia increases, unless the animal is receiving a cataleptic drug like ketamine. Rigid tone indicates inadequate depth of anesthesia.

b. *Cardiopulmonary function decreases with increasing depth of anesthesia.* As an animal becomes deeply anesthetized, respiration and cardiac output decrease. It results in poor blood oxygenation, tissue perfusion and decreased blood pressure. Likewise, elevations in the heart rate and blood pressure may be the indications that an animal may be feeling pain and is anesthetized too lightly.

c. There is also a reduction in *body temperature* with increase in the depth of anesthesia.

55. What types of anesthetics are preferred during retro-orbital blood collection from mice?

Ans: Proparacaine and tetracaine may be used as a local anesthetic during retro-orbital blood collection from mice. One drop is put in the eye and blood is withdrawn after 10–15 minutes.

56. What do you understand by term euthanasia in pharmacology?

Ans: Euthanasia means the sacrificing the animal in which there is rapid unconsciousness and subsequent death without or minimal pain or distress to animal.

57. Write down the different methods used for euthanasia.

Ans: Euthanasia methods are broadly classified as:

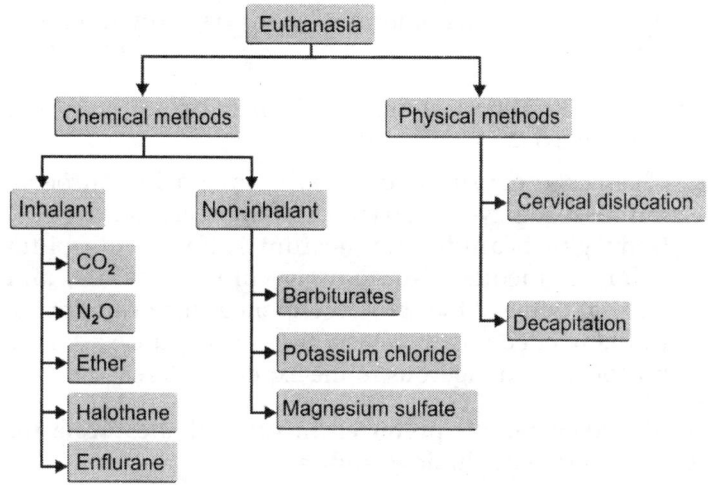

58. Write down the different ethically acceptable methods for different species used for euthanasia.

Ans:

Techniques	Acceptable	Not acceptable
Chemical		
Inhalant	• Carbon dioxide • Carbon dioxide plus halothane/chloroform • Carbon monoxide	• Ether • Argon flushing • Nitrogen flushing
Injectable	• Barbiturate overdose (IP) • Ketamine (IM/IP) • Sodium pentothol (IM/IP)	• Strychnine • Nicotine sulfate • Magnesium sulfate • Potassium chloride
Physical	• Cervical dislocation in rat, mouse and hamster • Decapitation in mouse and rat • Exsanguination in all except dog and monkey	• Decompression • Stunning • Rapid freezing • Asphyxia • Electrocution

(As per CPCSEA guidelines)

59. What are the physical methods which are not preferred for euthanasia?

Ans: Physical methods not to be used for euthanasia are exsanguination, rapid freezing, pithing, decompression, hyperthermia, hypothermia, asphyxia, drowning and strangulation.

60. What are the chemical methods which are not preferred for euthanasia?

Ans: Chemicals not to be used are carbon monoxide, nitrogen, nitrous oxide, cyclopropane, chloroform, trichloethylene, hydrogen cyanide, magnesium sulfate, potassium chloride, nicotine, strychnine, chloral hydrate, and ethanol. Some of the above mentioned chemicals are not recommended for euthanasia because they are extremely noxious and dangerous to the experimenter.

61. Which anesthetic is preferred in surgical anesthesia for CVS experiments in dogs and cats?

Ans: Chloralose

62. What is chloralose?

Ans: Chloralose is a compound of chloral and glucose prepared by heating equal parts of anhydrous glucose and chloral, when both α-chloralose (active form) and β-chloralose (inactive form) are formed. The hypnotic properties are limited to the α-isomer, i.e. α-chloralose (β-chloralose can result in muscular pain).

63. How is chloralose solution prepared?

Ans: Chloralose solution is prepared as 1% solution in 0.9% NaCl (saline) or in distilled water by heating to 60 °C, and administered intravenously or intraperitoneally at a temperature of 30 to 40 °C, before the chloralose comes out of solution. It is not very soluble in cold water, but is more soluble in hot water.

Alternatively, α-chloralose is heated in 100% PEG, keeping the temperature below 60 °C to prevent conversion to β-chloralose, which is non-anesthetic.

64. What is the effect of temperature on chloralose solution?

Ans: Heating of chloralose solution to above 60 °C causes decomposition. Its precipitation occurs at lower temperature (room temperature).

65. What are the advantages of chloralose as anesthetic?

Ans: It is a preferred anesthetic for cardiovascular experiments due to the following reasons:

a. Greater constancy of the depth of anesthesia.

b. Respiration and circulation are not depressed.

c. Blood pressure is well maintained.

d. Reflexes are not depressed.

66. What are the disadvantages of chloralose as an anesthetic?

Ans: a. Low water solubility and therefore, chloralose tends to precipitate at room temperature

b. Not suitable anesthetic for rabbits since the animals are narcotized rather than anesthetized

c. Large volume is needed

d. Animals may develop convulsions on slight stimulation

67. Which are preferred anesthetics in the models of pulmonary diseases?

Ans: Urethane (ethyl carbamate) is the most commonly employed anesthetic for pulmonary disease models. However, it disturbs thermoregulation. Therefore, anesthetized animals should be kept warm using a heating pad or lamp. Pentobarbital or ketamine disturbs the airway reflexes. Therefore, these should be avoided.

68. What are the disadvantages of urethane (ethyl carbamate) as an anaesthetic?

Ans: a. Used only for acute experiments

b. Delayed liver toxicity

c. Produce agranulocytosis

d. Produce pulmonary adenomata

e. Not suitable for mice as these develop high incidence of lung tumors

69. Why barbiturates are not preferred as anaesthetic for CVS studies?

Ans: Barbiturates produce cardiorespiratory depression and hypotension. Pentobarbitone has a strong vagolytic action, so it is not preferred for the evaluation of cardiovascular drugs.

ADVANCED TECHNIQUES USEFUL IN PHARMACOLOGY

70. What is patch clamp technique?

Ans: The patch clamp technique is an electrophysiological technique to study single or multiple ion channels in cells. The technique is applied to a wide variety of cells, but is especially useful in the study of excitable cells such as neurons, cardiomyocytes, muscle fibres and pancreatic beta cells. The patch clamp technique allows high-resolution recording of the ionic currents flowing through a single ion channel or whole cell's plasma membrane (Fig. 3.8).

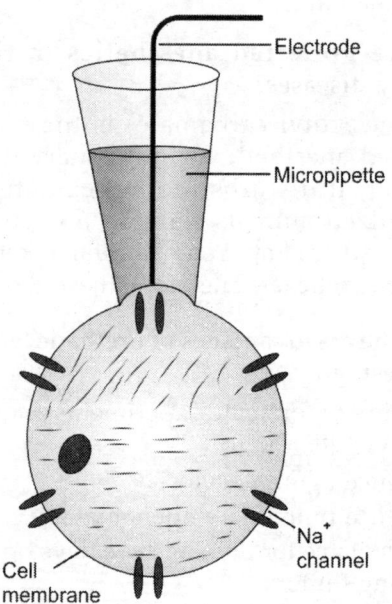

Fig. 3.8: Patch clamp technique for measuring the ionic currents

71. Who discovered patch clamp technique?

Ans: Erwin Neher and Bert Sakmann developed the patch clamp technique in the late 1970s and early 1980s and were awarded with Nobel Prize.

72. What are the various applications of the patch clamp technique?

Ans: The patch clamp technology has wide range of applications in the biology and in the basic medical research. It is used to study the functioning of single or multiple ion channels in a cell.

a. The effects on the excitability of cells due to non-functionality of these ion channels can be easily noted. There are numerous inherited diseases due to faulty channel function (ion channel mutation). Furthermore, in non-inherited diseases and tumors also, there is malfunctioning of definite ion channels or high expression of specific ion channels.

b. Patch clamp technique is used to evaluate the drugs that block/excite the ion channels.

c. The role of different ion channels in different diseases may be noted such as L-type voltage gated Ca^{2+} channel in cardiovascular research and stroke; voltage gated Na^+ channels in neuropathy.

d. Patch clamp recording on cultured and isolated cells is used to characterize the physiology and pharmacology of these channels, which play critical roles in several neurological disorders and other human diseases.

73. What are radio ligand binding studies?

Ans: A radio ligand is a radioactively labeled drug that can associate with a receptor (mostly), transporter or enzymes. The measurement of the rate and extent of binding of radio ligand with respect to test drug provide information on the number of binding sites and affinity of the test drug for that receptor.

74. Why we do radio ligand binding studies?

Ans: a. Receptors exist in very small concentrations in tissues. The most common method for detecting the receptors on membrane preparations and tissue is to use radioactive drugs, which have a high affinity and high degree of selectivity.

   b. The binding affinity of a new drug to a particular receptor may be noted using a radio ligand studies. During incubation of the tissue with radioactive drug under the appropriate experimental conditions, the radioactive drug (D) will bind to the receptor (R) to form a drug-receptor complex (RD). When the test drug is incubated with the drug-receptor complex, it shows displacement of radioactive ligand and radioactive ligand comes in supernatant.The extent of displacement of radio ligand drug denotes its affinity for the receptor.

   $$R + D^* \longrightarrow RD^*$$
   $$D_1 + RD^* \longrightarrow D_1R + D^*$$

   D^* is radioactive ligand and D_1 is at test drug.

75. What are the applications of radio ligand binding studies?

Ans: Radio ligand binding can be used to:

   a. characterize receptors in their natural environment.

   b. study receptor dynamics and localization.

   c. identify novel chemical structures that interact with the receptors.

   d. define ligand activity and selectivity in normal and diseased tissues.

76. What do you understand by dissociation constant?

Ans: Dissociation constant (K_i) of a test drug is the concentration at which 50% of receptors are occupied by test drug.

77. What is the significance of dissociation constant and how can it be calculated?

Ans: K_i determines the potency of drugs. The lower the value of K_i, the more potent is the drug and the drug is having more affinity for receptors.

$K_i = K_d \, [^3H] \times IC_{50}/Kd+[^3H]$

IC_{50} = concentration of test drug, which competes 50% of specifically bound drug in competition experiment

$[^3H]$ = concentration of labeled drug in the competition drug

$K_d \, [^3H]$ = dissociation constant of bound drug that is determined by saturation experiment

78. Name the different neurochemical techniques.

Ans: Different neurochemical techniques include histofluorescent technique, immunohistochemistry (immunocytochemistry), autoradiography, in situ hybridization and immunoassay techniques including radioimmunoassay.

79. What do you mean by immunohistochemistry?

Ans: Immunohistochemistry (IHC) combines anatomical, immunological and biochemical techniques to identify discrete tissue components (proteins in nature) by the interaction of target antigens with specific antibodies tagged with a visible label. IHC makes it possible to visualize the distribution and localization of specific protein components within tissues.

80. What is the utility of immunohistochemistry?

Ans: a. IHC is used for disease diagnosis, drug development and biological research. Using specific tumor markers, IHC is used to diagnose a cancer as benign or malignant, determine the stage and grade of a tumor, and identify the cell type and origin of a metastasis.

b. IHC is used in drug development to test the efficacy of test drug by detecting the up- or down-regulation of disease targets (protein components).

81. What is autoradiography?

Ans: Autoradiography is the mapping of the cellular components that have been radioactively labeled and it records the distribution of radioactive materials in histological specimens.

The first autoradiography was obtained accidently around 1867 when blackening was produced on emulsions of silver chloride and iodide by uranium salts.

82. What do you mean by *in situ* hybridization (ISH)?

Ans: ISH is a histochemical technique to localize specific nucleic acid sequence (DNA or RNA) in a portion or section of tissue (*in situ*). In this hybridization, a labeled complementary DNA or RNA strand (probe) is used to localize a specific DNA or RNA sequence in a section of tissue, the entire tissue (if it is small), and in cells (circulating tumor cells).

83. What are the applications of *in situ* hybridization (ISH) in neuropharmacology?

Ans: a. The sensitivity of the technique permits the detection of very small number of cells in CNS that express a particular gene, which otherwise could not be detected.

b. ISH identifies the population of cells that are actually capable of manufacturing a particular protein.

c. ISH may be used to identify the neuronal cells whose activity has been altered (temporary or adaptive changes in the form of neuronal plasticity) by environmental events or drugs.

d. Inherited neurological and neuropsychiatric disorders linked to abnormalities in the gene expression may also be evaluated by this technique.

84. What are radioimmunoassays (RIA)?

Ans: Radioimmunoassay (RIA) is an *in vitro* assay that measures the presence of an antigen with very high sensitivity using monoclonal antibodies labeled with radioactive material. Basically any biological substance for which a specific antibody exists can be measured, even in minute concentrations. RIA has been the first immunoassay technique developed to analyze nanomolar and picomolar concentrations of hormones in biological fluids.

In vitro Experiments

4

FOR UNDERGRADUATES AND POSTGRADUATES

1. What do you understand by *in vitro*?

Ans: In pharmacology, it is the experimental process which is done outside the living body using isolated tissue preparation, isolated cells and enzymes.

2. What do you understand by *ex vivo*?

Ans: It is the experimental process which is performed outside the living body in an artificial *in vivo* environment.

3. What do you understand by *in vivo*?

Ans: It is the experimental process which is mainly done inside the living body, e.g. pharmacodynamics or pharmacokinetic study of drugs.

4. What do you understand by *in situ*?

Ans: It means to measure the function of an organ at the same anatomical position (mainly done in anesthetized or sacrificed animals).

5. What do you understand by *in silico*?

Ans: It is the experimental process which is performed on computer or via computer stimulations.

6. What do you understand by the term DRC?

Ans: DRC stands for dose-response curve which represents a simple X-Y graph relating the amount of a drug to the response of the receptor. DRC demonstrates graded responses to drugs or agonists where an increase in response is recorded with a subsequent increase in the dose or the concentration of the drug. The typical DRC is sigmoid or S-shaped (Fig. 4.1).

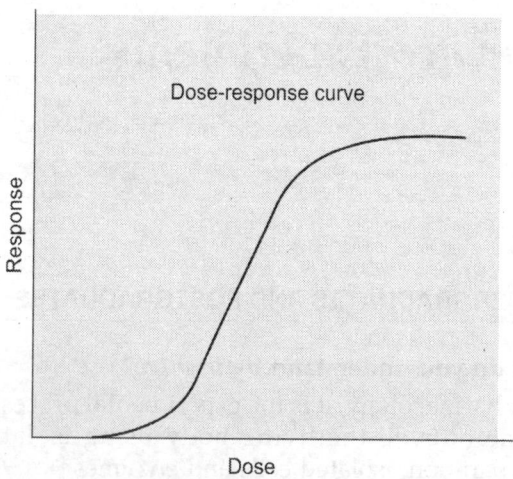

Fig. 4.1: Dose-response curve (DRC)

7. **What do you understand by term cumulative dose-response curve?**

Ans: The cumulative dose-response curve is obtained by increasing the concentration of drug in an organ bath step by step without washing the preceding doses. In this way, the drug is cumulated in the organ bath and response is increased.

8. **What is the difference between cumulative dose-response curve (CRC) and dose-response curve (DRC)?**

Ans: In CRC, curve is obtained by increasing the concentration of drug in the organ bath step by step without washing the preceding doses, whereas in DRC, curve is obtained by increasing the concentration of drug in the organ bath step by step with washing out the preceding doses (previously added doses).

9. **What are the advantages of cumulative dose-response curve?**

Ans: The technique is simple and less time consuming.

10. Where is cumulative dose-response curve used?

Ans: It is generally employed in those preparations where the tissue is slow contracting and slow relaxing. *Example*: response curve of angiotensin using rat aortic muscle.

11. Where is cumulative dose-response curve not used?

Ans: This method is not suited for drugs which show "fade phenomenon", i.e. the response of the drug tend to decrease of its own without washing the drug, e.g. uterus preparation.

12. What is the difference between arithmetic and geometric addition?

Ans: In arithmetic addition, doses are added in arithmetic progression, i.e. 1, 2, 3, 4, 5, 6, ..., whereas in geometric addition, the doses are added in geometric progression, i.e. 1, 2, 4, 8, 16, 32, ..., etc.

13. In which manner doses are added to plot DRC?

Ans: For the convenience of plotting the dose-response curve, the doses are increased in geometric progression (logarithmic intervals).

14. Why doses are added in geometric progression to plot DRC?

Ans: The doses are added in geometric progression due to the following reasons:

a. The geometric doses represent log doses and biological responses are linear to log doses. Therefore, the progression in the response during geometric addition is nearly linear.

b. More dose range may be covered using lesser number of doses.

15. What does DRC indicate?

Ans: The following important parameters may be deduced from DRC

- *Relative potency of the drug or agonist*: When the curve is more towards the left, it indicates that the drug is more potent.

- *Error and reliability (precision)*: It is indicated by slope of the curve. The steeper the curve, more precise is the assay and vice versa.
- *Efficacy of the drug*: It is indicated by maximum response of the curve. Higher the maximal response, higher is the efficacy (Fig. 4.2).

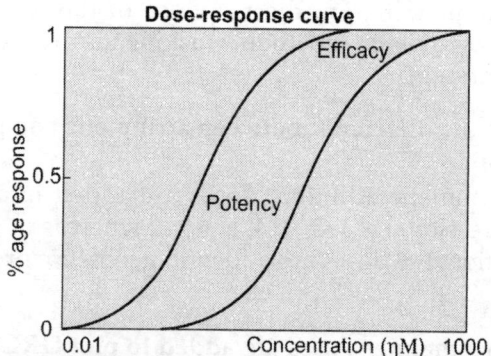

Fig. 4.2: Dose-response curve (DRC) representing potency, precision and efficacy of drug

16. **What is the advantage of log dose-response curve over dose-response curve?**

Ans: Generally, log dose-response is preferred over dose-response curve because biological responses are directly proportional to log doses. Therefore, the following advantages are offered:

    a. The linear portion of the sigmoid curve becomes straighter.

    b. Comparison of two dose-response curves is much simpler.

    c. Large dose ranges can be plotted which is otherwise difficult in dose-response curves.

    d. The error is distributed all through the graph, independent of the dose.

17. **What do you understand by ED$_{50}$?**

Ans: ED$_{50}$ is a dose or concentration producing 50% of maximal response. Lower the value more potent is the drug (Fig. 4.3).

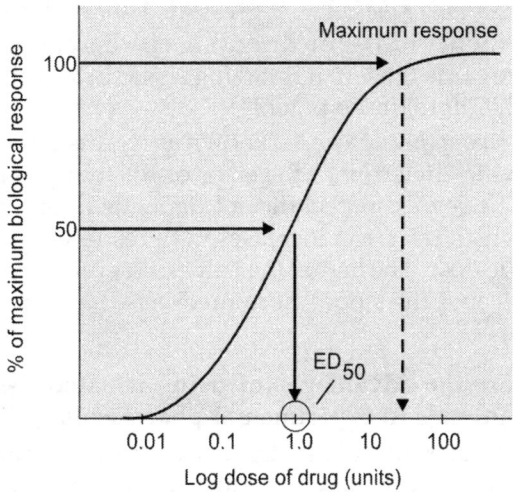

Fig. 4.3: ED_{50}: Median effective dose

18. What is isometric recording?

Ans: In this type of recording, the muscle length is held constant and force developed due to contraction of muscle is translated into force, which is recorded.

19. What is isotonic recording?

Ans: In this type of recording, the contractile tissue (muscle) is allowed to shorten against a constant load.

20. What is axotonic recording?

Ans: In reality, muscles rarely contract under strictly isometric or isotonic conditions. In this type of recordings, the tension in the muscle increases with shortening of muscle.

21. What are the different parameters that are characterized by dose response curve?

Ans: a. *Maximal or ceiling effect*: Commonly referred to E_{max} or efficacy. Maximum effect is different from potency. Different efficacies suggest different mechanisms of drug.

b. *Position of the curve*: It gives idea about the affinity or potency, ED_{50} of drug, e.g. if the curve is more towards the left, it is having lesser ED_{50} value, and is therefore, more potent.

c. *Slope of the curve*: Also known as regression coefficient, which determines the error or reliability of an assay. The regression coefficient depends upon the rate at which the effect increases with respect to increase in the dose. The higher the value of regression coefficient steeper the slope, more precise is the assay and vice versa.

22. What are the advantages of using isolated tissue over intact animals in experimental pharmacology?

Ans: Advantages of isolated tissue over intact animals are:

a. Several preparations can be obtained from a single animal as generally and relatively small amount of test material is required for pharmacological testing.

b. The effects of drugs are tested directly without the interference of drug absorption, metabolism, excretion or interference due to nerve reflexes.

c. It requires usage of very less amount of test drug (which is very expensive many times).

d. The antagonistic or potentiating effects of drugs can be easily elucidated in isolated tissue preparations than in intact animals.

23. What are the common sources of isolated tissue?

Ans: Rats, rabbits and Guinea pig are usually the common sources of isolated tissues. Mice are also sometime used, while cats and dogs are too big to sacrifice just for a piece of tissue.

24. What is the most commonly employed smooth muscle preparation for *in vitro* testing?

Ans: Intestine is the most commonly employed smooth muscle preparations because of the following reasons:

a. It provides abundant tissue for testing.

b. It is relatively more resistant to handling.

c. It is relatively easy to set up.

d. It permits the study of different types of pharmacological actions as there are very large number of receptors localized on intestine.

e. Amongst the different portions of intestine, ileum is more preferred because it produces larger contraction than jejunum or duodenum.

25. What are the main components of physiological salt solution (PSS)?

Ans: Main components of PSS are sodium (Na^+), potassium (K^+), chloride (Cl^-), magnesium (Mg^+), calcium (Ca^{2+}) and glucose.

26. What is the significance of these main components in PSS?

Ans: *Sodium* (Na^+): It is a major extracellular cation and makes the solution isotonic by maintaining the osmolarity.

Potassium (K^+): It is a major intracellular cation and is very important for nerve conduction, and muscle contraction. It is also important in maintaining the heart rate and rhythm.

Calcium chloride ($CaCl_2$): It controls the excitability of muscles and nerves. It is an essential component for muscle contraction.

Magnesium chloride ($MgCl_2$): It is the second most common intracellular cation. Its major action is to reduce the spontaneous activity of tissue. It also controls the neurotransmission in muscle contraction.

27. What are the precautions to be taken during PSS preparation?

Ans: PSS should always be prepared in distilled or deionizer water, otherwise there will be salting out of the dissolved components. Calcium chloride solution should be made separately and is to be added in rest of solution at last. Aeration is important for PSS and it has to be done using carbogen (95% O_2 + 5% CO_2). Pure O_2 may interact with HCO_3 in PSS, which will cause CO_2 loss and PSS becomes alkaline.

28. **Why calcium chloride should be added at last while making PSS?**

Ans: The solution of calcium chloride should be made separately and should be added in rest of solution at last to prevent precipitation or chelation of bicarbonate, which makes solution turbid.

29. **Why is drug concentration expressed in molar concentration?**

Ans: a. By expressing the concentration in molar units, it is not necessary to specify the nature of the salt used. For example, acetylcholine chloride and acetylcholine bromide, there is no need to tell the salt form.

b. Comparison between results obtained by different workers become easier and more rational.

c. It is the active mass of the drug rather than the actual weight of whole salt that is more important in drug action, e.g. it is the acetylcholine which is biologically active not chloride or bromide.

30. **Who designed the assembly for recording of contraction of isolated tissues?**

Ans: Rudolph Magnus was first to design the arrangement of bath for excised organs (intestinal strips) as early as in 1904.

31. **Why is aeration necessary for isolated tissue preparations?**

Ans: Aeration has dual function in isolated tissue preparations. It not only provides oxygen to tissue, but also stirs the bath solution to facilitate the diffusion of drug added to the bath.

32. **What do you understand by the term magnification?**

Ans: Magnification is defined as the ratio of distance from fulcrum to writing point to distance from fulcrum to tied tissue. In plotting DRC of isolated muscle preparation, the contraction of muscle is magnified and plotted on a paper. The magnification has to be varied depending on the type of muscle, i.e. feeble contracting muscle or strong contracting muscle (Fig. 4.4).

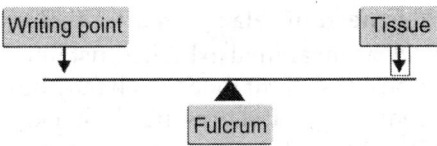

Fig. 4.4: Magnification: Ratio of distance from fulcrum to writing point to distance from fulcrum to tied tissue

33. What is the speed of the drum used in recordings?

Ans: For most of the experiments, a speed of one revolution in 96 minutes is usually used.

34. What are the different types of writing levers used in recordings?

Ans: Two types of levers are used in isolated tissue preparations (Fig. 4.5).

Class Type I: The fulcrum or pivot lies between the writing point and the point of attachment of the tissue.

Class Type II: The fulcrum lies at the one end beyond the point of attachment.

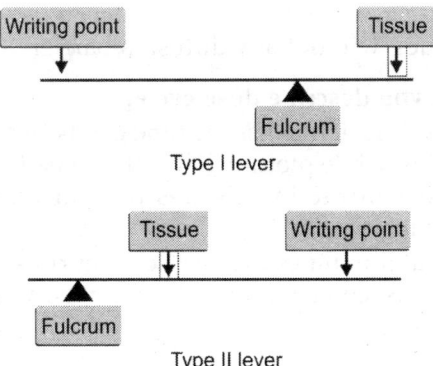

Fig. 4.5: Different types of writing levers used in recordings

35. Why there is need of relaxation after isolation of tissue?

Ans: The muscle from animal exhibit a sustained submaximal contraction or inherent tone which may be of neurogenic or myogenic origin. It represents the background activity of muscle. When the animal is sacrificed the degree of muscle tone is further increased. Therefore, if response reading is taken immediately after mounting the tissue in an organ tube, the smooth muscle tissues may respond by relaxation (rather than contraction) following addition of particular drug.

36. What are the slow contracting tissue/muscles?

Ans: Frog rectus abdominus muscle, stomach fundus, biventer cervices muscle of chick, Guinea pig tracheal smooth muscle, etc.

37. What are the fast contracting tissue/muscles?

Ans: Fast contracting tissue/muscles are ileum, uterus, ascending and descending colon, etc.

38. What do you understand by the term Biophase?

Ans: The environment in which drug is free to interact with receptors without any intervening diffusion barriers is called biophase. In isolated tissue preparations, the tissue is mounted in the inner organ tube (filled with physiological salt solution) and therefore, represents the biophase in which drug is free to act on receptors located on tissues, without any diffusion barrier.

39. How can you describe dose cycle?

Ans: Dose cycle is defined as the time gap between drug dose additions, while plotting DRC. It is usually of 3 minutes for fast contracting tissues or 5 minutes for slow contracting tissues.
A typical 5 minutes dose cycle comprises a baseline of 30 seconds, contact time of 90 seconds, and 3 washings of 1 minute.

40. How can you describe contact time?

Ans: It is defined as the time duration during which tissue comes in contact with drug. Usually, a contact time of 90 seconds is chosen for slow contracting muscles.

41. What do you understand by sensitivity?

Ans: It has different definitions with respect to different contexts. For bioassays, it is the minimum amount of drug which is able to produce a biological response. For a given drug, the sensitivity will vary depending upon the tissue. The tissue which responds to minimum amount of drug is said to be the most sensitive tissue for that particular drug.

42. What are the different stages in oestrous cycle?

Ans: There are four stages in four-day oestrous cycle. These include proestrus followed by frankestrus (estrus), metaestrus and diestrus. The mating usually takes place on the night between the days of proestrus and frankestrus.

43. What are the microscopic features of vaginal smear in these different stages of oestrous cycle?

Ans: The vaginal smear of four stages of oestrous cycle, i.e. proestrus, frank estrus (estrus), metaestrus and diestrus are differentiated mainly by presence of cells which are predominant in smear.

S. No.	Stage	Epithelial cells	Cornified epithelial cells	Leukocytes
1.	Proestrus	+++	++	±
2.	Frankestrus (estrus)	±	+++	–
3.	Metaestrus	++	±	+++
4.	Diestrus	+	+	+++

44. How can you differentiate these cells under light microscope without staining?

Ans: Cornified epithelial cells are irregular (horny) in shape, nuclei is absent and generally dark due to deposition of keratin. The epithelial cells are round to oval shaped, relatively larger in size than neutrophils. Neutrophils are very small round shaped cells (Figs. 4.6 a and b).

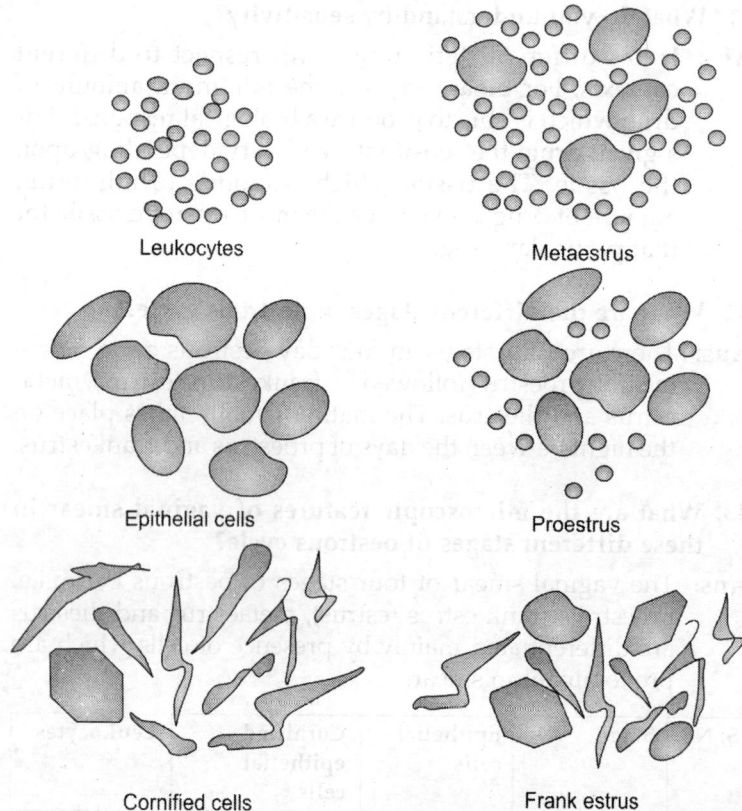

Leukocytes   Metaestrus

Epithelial cells   Proestrus

Cornified cells   Frank estrus

Figs 4.6a and b: Different stages including diestrus, proestrus, and frank estrus differentiated on the basis of presence of leukocytes, epithelial cells and cornified epithelial cells under light microscope

45. **In which, the uterus is most sensitive to oxytocin?**

Ans: Frank estrus stage.

46. **How can frank estrus stage be induced in rats before isolating uterus for obtaining DRC?**

Ans: Administration of stilboestrol (0.1 ml/kg) subcutaneously may induce frank estrus stage which can assessed by taking vaginal smear 24 hours after stilboestrol injection. It is a usual procedure to inject stilboestrol (0.1 ml/kg)

24 hours before isolating the uterus preparation so that uterus is in frank estrus stage, the most sensitive stage.

47. What is the relevance of using isolated uterine preparation?

Ans: One of the relevance is screening of potential uterine contracting agents as anti-fertility or abortifacients agents and uterine relaxants as tocolytics.

48. What is the physiological solution used in rat uterus preparation?

Ans: De Jalon's solution

49. What is the major difference between De Jalon and Ringer-Locke's solutions?

Ans: The composition of both salt solutions is same except that De Jalon's solution contains one-fourth amount of $CaCl_2$ and half amount of glucose.

50. What is the optimum temperature employed in rat uterus preparation?

Ans: About 30 °C

51. How may the sensitivity of rat uterus be increased?

Ans: The sensitivity of rat uterus to oxytocin may be increased by:

a. Superfusion technique

b. Taking uterus from rat in frank estrus stage

c. Elimination of Mg^{2+} from the bath solution also increases the sensitivity

52. What is the effect of pH on uterine spontaneity?

Ans: The decrease in pH decreases the spontaneous contraction of uterus. Accordingly, to reduce spontaneous contraction the pH may be lowered by aerating with oxygen containing 5% CO_2.

53. What is the load and magnification for isolated uterus preparation?

Ans: The load on a lever is about 0.5 gm and magnification is about 5–10 folds.

54. How does the response obtained in uterus is different from fundus and ileum?

Ans: The responses obtained in uterus are quicker than those produced by fundus. But these are slower as compared to that of ileum. Furthermore, response in uterus is not sustained and tissue partly relaxes, while drug is still present in the bath (fade phenomenon).

55. What is the use of rat stomach preparation in drug evaluation?

Ans: Rat's stomach is most suitable preparation for the assay of 5-hydroxytryptamine because it is very sensitive to serotonin (about 10 times more sensitive to acetylcholine).

56. How does a fundus is differentiated from pyloric region of stomach?

Ans: The fundus part is grey in color and pyloric part is pinkish in color in rat stomach.

57. What is the magnification and load used in isolated fundus preparation?

Ans: The load in horizontal position is usually 1 gm and magnification may as high as 16. However, usually magnification of 5–7 may be used.

58. Why is the relevance of using frog rectus abdominus muscle?

Ans: Rectus abdominus muscle of frog is a perfect skeletal muscle for *in vitro* experimentation. It is rich in nicotinic receptors and responds to acetylcholine. It is used for the assay of acetylcholine as well as tubocurarine like drugs (skeletal muscle relaxants).

59. What are the special precautions that should be taken during isolation of rectus abdominus?

Ans: Generally, blood vessels run along the back of rectus abdominus. It is important that these blood vessels should be removed or at least blood present in these muscles should be removed. Otherwise, due to presence of cholinesterase enzyme, the acetylcholine will be degraded and there will be no response of acetylcholine.

60. What is the main characteristic feature of rectus abdominis muscle that makes it useful preparation for plotting DRC?

Ans: Frog rectus abdominis muscle is a voluntary muscle preparation (skeletal muscle). Unlike other skeletal muscle preparations (skeletal muscles usually give a twitch response), it produces slow contraction and slow relaxation (a characteristic feature of smooth muscle) in response to exogenous acetylcholine administration.

FOR POSTGRADUATES

61. What are the different experimental methods of determining the competitive nature of antagonism?

Ans: The following methods are generally employed to determine the type of antagonism:
- *Parallel shift of the concentration-response curve*: The right hand parallel shift of a dose-response curve indicates the competitive antagonism.
- *Double reciprocal plot of Lineweaver – Burk*: If the straight lines determined in the presence or absence of the antagonist, intersect on the line corresponding to infinite dose, the antagonism is said to be competitive (Fig. 4.7).

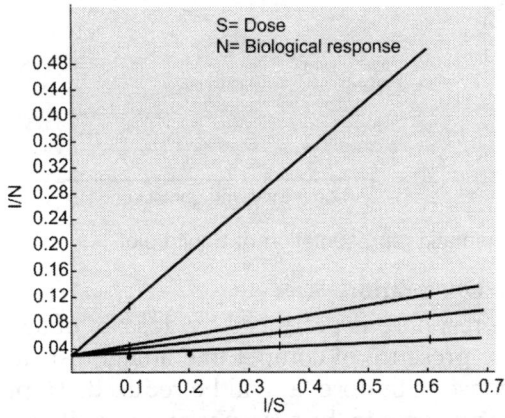

Fig. 4.7: Schematic representation of Lineweaver – Burk plot

- *Schild plot*: A plot with a slope very near to unity signifies the competitive antagonism.
- *Difference between pA_2 and pA_{10} values*: If the difference between pA_2 and pA_{10} values is in the range of 0.8–1.2 (near to 0.95), then antagonism is competitive in nature.

62. Define pA_2 values.

Ans: The pA_2 value is defined as the negative logarithm of the molar concentration of antagonist that makes it necessary to double the concentration of agonist to elicit the original submaximal response.

63. What is Schild plot?

Ans: Schild plot is a commonly used method for estimating pA_2 values. In fact it is a graph plotted between log (DR-1) and negative log (I). DR represents the agonist dose-ratio and (I) represents the molar concentration of the antagonist. When the Schild plot gives a straight line with a slope which is near to unity, then antagonism is competitive (Fig. 4.8).

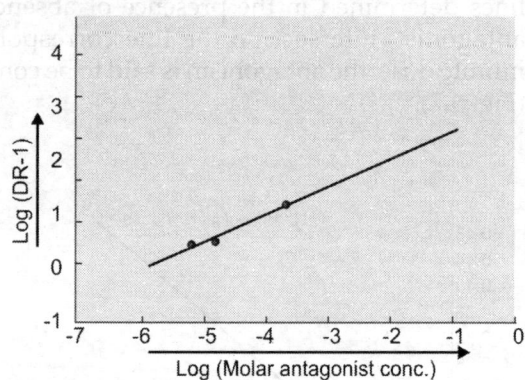

Fig. 4.8: Schematic representation of Schild plot

64. Define Dose ratio.

Ans: Let a response is produced by dose 'a' of agonist. Now in the presence of competitive antagonist (dose B), the response with dose 'a' will be reduced. To produce the same response in the presence of competitive antagonist, the dose of agonist has to be increased from 'a' to 'A'. This ratio A/a is called dose ratio.

Where,

A = amount of agonist required to produce a 'defined response' in the presence of a competitive antagonist with dose B

a = amount of agonist required to produce a 'defined response' in the absence of an antagonist

65. What is the affinity constant of antagonist for receptors?

Ans: Let 'B' = amount of antagonist; 'a' have meaning explained earlier, then

$A/a = 1+B\,K_B$

K_B = affinity constant for antagonist

66. Define pA_2 in terms of dose ratio and affinity constant.

Ans: As $A/a = 1+B\,K_B$ dose ratio = 2 for pA_2

$2 = 1 + B\,K_B,$

$1 = B\,K_B$

$K_B = 1/B;$

$\log K_B = \log 1/B$

Because, $\log 1/B = pA_2;$ therefore $pA_2 = \log K_B$

67. What is the significance of calculating pA_2 and pA_{10} values?

Ans: A method of testing competitive or noncompetitive nature of an antagonist is to determine both pA_2 and pA_{10} values for the agonist-antagonist pair on the same tissue. If the difference between these two values is found to be 0.95 or very near (0.8–1.2), the antagonism is likely to be competitive.

These two pA values may be calculated from the Schild plot line and the difference is calculated. A value which is very different from 0.95 suggests that inhibition is not competitive.

68. What is Lineweaver and Burk plot?

Ans: In Lineweaver and Burk plot, the reciprocal of the biological response is plotted against the reciprocal of the dose. If the points lie on straight lines, and if the straight lines determined in the presence or absence of the antagonist, intersect on the line corresponding to infinite dose, the antagonism is said to be competitive.

69. **What are the isolated tissues employed for evaluating α_1- adrenoreceptors?**

Ans: *Guinea pig atria:*
Agonist: Isoproterenol, dobutamine
Antagonist: Atenolol

70. **What are the isolated tissues employed to evaluate α_2- adrenoreceptors?**

Ans: a. Guinea pig tracheal smooth muscle
Agonist: Salbutamol
Antagonist: Propranolol
 b. Rat uterus preparation

71. **For what purpose isolated vas deferens muscle is employed?**

Ans: Isolated vas deferens muscle is employed for studying α_1-adrenorecepton subtypes as this muscle responds to noradrenergic agents.

72. **What are the other isolated tissues that are employed for evaluating α_1-adrenoreceptors?**

Ans: Rat spleen and isolated rat aorta

73. **What are the models of urinary urge incontinence?**

Ans: Measurement of pelvic nerve stimulated urinary bladder contraction in rats/dogs.

74. **How do skeletal muscle relaxants (peripherally acting) are assayed?**

Ans: Neuromuscular blockers are typically assayed by employing skeletal muscles of the following types:
 a. Isolated rectus abdominis muscle of frog
 b. Isolated phrenic nerve—diaphragm preparation of rat

75. **What are the different tests for evaluating neuromuscular blocking activity?**

Ans: a. Rabbit sciatic nerve—gastrocnemius muscle preparation
 b. Isolated phrenic nerve—diaphragm preparation of rat
 c. Chick sciatic nerve—tibialis anticus muscle preparation

76. What is the limitation of isolated phrenic nerve diaphragm preparation?

Ans: It is an excellent method for determining the potency of drug to block or facilitate neuromuscular transmission. However using this preparation, it is not possible to distinguish between depolarizing and non-depolarizing neuromuscular blocking agent. In this situation, chick sciatic nerve libialis anticus muscle preparation is preferred.

77. How are cysteinyl leukotriene receptor assays performed in isolated tissues?

Ans: Cysteinyl leukotrienes (LTC_4, LTD_4 and LTE_4) are lipid products derived from arachidonic acid metabolism. These leukotrienes are involved in the development of asthma as these produces potent bronchoconstriction. Cysteinyl leukotrienes are assayed by noting smooth muscle contraction using Guinea pig trachea.

78. What are the different tissues employed for 5-hydroxy-tryptamine receptor assay?

Ans:

Receptors	Tissues and Response
$5\text{-}HT_{1A}$	Inhibition of twitch response in transmurally electrically stimulated Guinea pig ileum
$5\text{-}HT_{1B}$	Contraction of rat caudal artery
$5\text{-}HT_{1D}$	• Relaxation of precontracted Guinea pig jugular vein • Contraction of rabbit cerebral arteries
$5\text{-}HT_{2A}$	Contraction of rabbit thoracic aorta
$5\text{-}HT_{2B}$	Contraction of rat stomach fundus
$5\text{-}HT_{2C}$	Contraction of rat jugular vein
$5\text{-}HT_3$	Contraction of Guinea pig ilea smooth muscle
$5\text{-}HT_4$	Relaxation of rat esophageal tunica muscularis mucosa
$5\text{-}HT_7$	Relaxation of endothelium denuded precontracted rabbit jugular vein

79. What is the effect of Tyrode's solution on uterus preparation?

Ans: Tyrode's solution is unfavorable medium for isolated uterus and it tends to render the uterus inactive and inresponsive.

80. How does spontaneous activity of uterus change with time?

Ans: The spontaneous activity of isolated uterus varies with time. When first set up, most preparations show marked activity and high sensitivity for a short-while. However, the activity tend to decreases over first hour and then become stable for 1–3 hours.

81. What do you understand by Gaddum's technique of superfusion?

Ans: In this technique, uterus is superfused by oxytocin, i.e. oxytocin is added dropwise from upward direction. It increases the sensitivity of rat uterus. It becomes sensitive to as little as to oxytocin in 0.3 ml and gives more reliable response than a uterus maintained in an isolated organ bath.

82. Write the drugs that may be used to plot DRC of rat fundus strip along with their sensitivity?

Ans:

Sr. No.	Drugs	Doses	Volume
1.	5-HT (serotonin)	10^{-7} M	0.1 ml
2.	Acetylcholine	10^{-6} M	0.1 ml
3.	Nicotine	10^{-3} M	0.1 ml
4.	Histamine	10^{-3} M	0.1 ml

Nicotine produces complex response and it may produce a relaxation followed by a contraction. Histamine also produces feeble contractions.

83. What is the characteristics feature of chick biventer cervicis preparation?

Ans: This is the muscle present behind the neck (back of neck) of chick. There are two biventer cervicis muscles present on either side of midline.

The special feature of this muscle is that it contains both slow and twitch fibres. It gives twitch responses, similar to those obtained with rat diaphragm, when stimulated electrically. However, it also gives slow contraction, similar to rectus abdominus, when acetylcholine drug is added.

84. What is the difference in doses of acetylcholine used in chick biventer cervicis and rectus abdominus?

Ans: For chick biventer cervicis preparation, relatively high dose of acetylcholine is used. This is due to presence of large amount of very active cholinesterase enzyme present in the muscle.

85. What is the problem of fundus muscle relaxation during plotting DRC?

Ans: Sometimes, this muscle does not relax spontaneously after it has been contracted by adding drug. This can be resolved by adding 1 gm of extra load to stretch it downwards for its relaxation.

86. What are special precautions that should be taken while stretching the smooth muscle for relaxation?

Ans: a. The muscle should only be stretched only if muscle does not relax spontaneously even after washing for 3–4 times.

b. Since the fundus is a smooth muscle, it should not be stretched too much. Very high stretching may destroy the smooth muscle.

87. What type of lever may be preferred for isolated fundus preparation?

Ans: It is better to use auxotonic lever. In this type, the load increases as muscle contracts and shortens. So it avoids the use of extra load and stretching during relaxation phase.

88. When should a new dose of drug be added after muscle is relaxed after stretching?

Ans: If muscle is stretched for its relaxation, then extra time of at least 4–5 minutes should be given before adding a new drug.

89. How does the uterus respond to adrenaline, noradrenaline and isoprenaline?

Ans: Isolated uterus is insensitive to noradrenaline. However, it is quite sensitive to adrenaline and isoprenaline. So it may be very useful to assay adrenaline in a mixture containing noradrenaline.

90. How many uterus preparations may be isolated from a single rat?

Ans: From a single rat, two horns of uterus are removed. Each horn is divided longitudinally. So four pieces are obtained from each animal.

91. Give example of tissues for which cumulative response curve may be obtained.

Ans: The aortic strip of rat responds very slowly and takes a long time to recover. Therefore, for evaluating angiotensin receptor modulators (agonists and antagonists), CRC may be plotted. Angiotensin II and agonists produce contraction of aorta.

92. What are the different blood coagulation tests?

Ans: Blood coagulation tests include prothrombin time (PT), activated partial thromboplastin time (aPTT) and thrombin time (TT) tests.

93. How can prothrombin time (PT) be determined?

Ans: An aliquot of 0.1 ml of citrated plasma is incubated for 1 minute at 37 °C, then 0.2 ml of human thromboplastin is added and time to clot formation is determined. An abnormal prothrombin time is often caused by liver disease or injury or by treatment with blood warfarin like drugs.

94. What does prothrombin time (PT) indicate?

Ans: The PT measures the integrity of the exogenous pathway in which there is release of thromboplastin (tissue factor) leading to activation of factor VII. The normal PT time is 12–14 seconds and it is normally used to monitor the drug therapy of warfarin.

95. How can activated partial thromboplastin time (aPTT) be determined?

Ans: To 0.1 ml of citrated plasma, 0.1 ml of human placenta lipid extract (or negatively charged phospholipid, lipid and kaolin) is added and the mixture is incubated for 2 minutes at 37 °C. The coagulation process is initiated by the addition of 0.1 ml 25 mM calcium chloride and time to clot formation is determined. The aPTT measures the integrity of intrinsic pathway of coagulation.

96. What does activated partial thromboplastin time (aPTT) indicate?

Ans: The aPTT measures the effects on the intrinsic pathway via factors XII, XI and IX to activation of factor VII. The normal aPTT time is 26–33 seconds and it is normally used to monitor the drug therapy of heparin (kept at 50–80 seconds).

97. How can thrombin time (TT) be determined?

Ans: To 0.1 ml of citrated plasma 0.1 ml of diethylbarbiturate-citrate buffer, pH 7.6 is added and the mixture is incubated for 1 minute at 37 °C. Then 0.1 ml of bovine test—thrombin is added and time to clot formation is determined. The TT measures effect on fibrin formation.

98. What is euglobulin lysis?

Ans: Euglobulin predominantly consists of plasmin, plasminogen, plasminogen activator and fibrinogen. By addition of thrombin to this fraction, fibrin clots are formed. The lysis time of these clots is determined as a measurement of the activity of activators of fibrinolysis (e.g. plasminogen activators). Thus, compounds which stimulate the release of tissue-type plasminogen activator from the vessel wall promote euglobulin lysis.

99. What does euglobulin lysis time indicate?

Ans: The euglobulin lysis time is used to evaluate the drugs that influence the fibrinolytic activity in blood.

100. Differentiate between perfusion and infusion.

Ans: A perfusion is a process in which there is a provision of inward flow of fluid as well as outward flow of fluid. Incoming fluid provides nourishment to tissue and outflowing fluid removes the waste material from tissue. On the other hand, during infusion, only consideration is made on introduction of fluid and it is similar to injection of fluid. Infusion means introduction of a solution into the body through a vein for therapeutic purpose (Fig. 4.9).

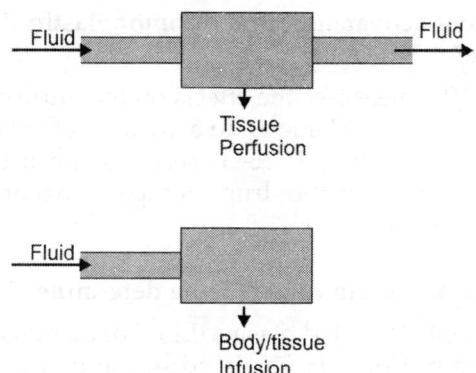

Fig. 4.9: Schematic representation of perfusion and infusion

101. What is *Langendroff*?

Ans: In 1897, *Oscar Langendroff* established the isolated perfusion mammalian heart preparation, which is considered as major breakthrough in cardiovascular research (Fig. 4.10).

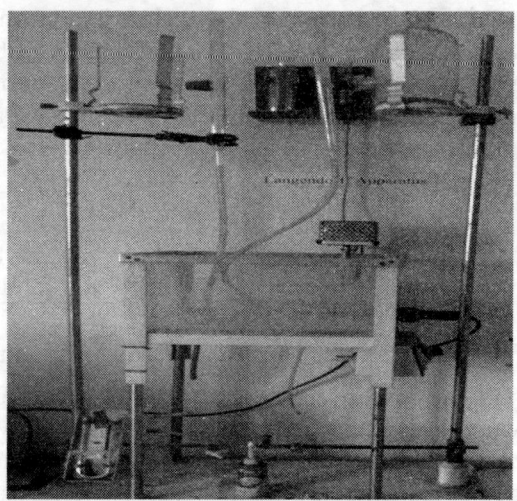

Fig. 4.10: Langendroff's apparatus for isolated rat heart perfusion

102. What is the basic principle in Langendroff's heart preparation?

Ans: The principle is based on the retrograde flow in the aorta either at constant flow or constant pressure. The physiological solution is allowed to enter the coronary arteries from the aortia. The physiological salt solution passes through the coronary circulation and then perfusate drains into the right atrium via the coronary sinus.

103. How can be the injury minimized to heart while mounting on the Langendroff's system?

Ans: Transfer of isolated heart immediately to ice cold physiological salt solution reduces the metabolic activity as well as beating which results in low requirement of glucose and oxygen. This minimizes the injury to heart before/and during mounting on Langendorff's system.

104. What do you understand by Hypodynamic heart?

Ans: Hypodynamic heart is defined as the heart exhibiting subnormal power or force than the normal one. Experimentally, it is developed by the supply of 1/4th of calcium chloride ($CaCl_2$) than the required one which reduces the heart.

5

In vivo Experiments

FOR UNDERGRADUATES AND POSTGRADUATES

1. **What are the different tests to evaluate sedative and hypnotic activity of a drug? Which is the most preferred test for the same?**

Ans: a. Loss of righting reflex
   b. Barbiturate sleeping time
   c. Potentiation of anesthesia
   d. Determination of 'motor activity' using photo cell method.
   Photo cell counter method is the most preferred method in rats and mice.

2. **What is MES model?**

Ans: MES stands for maximal electroshock model in which high intensity shocks are applied to the head of a rodent to produce tonic-clonic convulsions. Maximal electroshock model is used to evaluate the drugs used for the treatment of grand mal epilepsy. The antiepileptic drugs inhibit the tonic hind limb extension phase of epilepsy in MES model.

3. **What kind of substances/drugs can be screened by maximal electroshock (MES) test?**

Ans: It is used to screen the chemical substances that prevent the spread of electric discharge through the neural tissues in CNS and protect against maximal shock-induced seizure. The drugs effective in grand mal epilepsy (generalized tonic-clonic convulsions) are generally evaluated using this model. These drugs effectively inhibit the tonic phase (especially extensor phase) of convulsions.

4. **Why we use Rota rod test?**

Ans: Rota rod test is used to evaluate the fore and hind limb motor co-ordination of rodents. Retention time of each mouse/rat on the revolving rod is recorded. It is mainly employed to assess the muscle strength of an animal. The drugs that produce skeletal muscle relaxation are usually evaluated using rota rod test. The "Rota rod" technique is essential in screening drugs which have side effects on motor co-ordination.

5. **What are the different types of pain?**

Ans: Pain is generally classified into two types: Nociceptive pain and neuropathic pain. Nociceptive pain occurs when there is some damage/injury to tissue and ceases to occur once the injury is healed. On the other hand, neuropathic pain occurs when there is injury to a nerve and pain persists despite the tissue healing.

6. **What are the different nociceptive tests performed to assess nociceptive pain in animals?**

Ans: The nociception may be evaluated in animals by tail flick test, tail immersion test, writhing test and eddy's hot plate test.

7. **Who developed the tail flick procedure for testing analgesics?**

Ans: The tail flick procedure was developed by D'Armour and Smith in 1941 for both rats and mice.

8. **What are the precautions that should be taken while holding the animal for tail flick testing?**

Ans: The animal should not be held too tightly so that it cannot flick the tail. Furthermore, the head portion (including eyes) should be covered with cloth to prevent visualization mediated interference with the flick of tail.

9. **What is the nature of pain receptors?**

Ans: Pain receptors are free nerve endings terminating on the skin.

10. What are the nerve fibers that transmit pain?

Ans: There are three types of nerve fibers

  C fibers: These are thin (0.4 ± 1.2 mm in diameter), unmyelinated and slowly conducting (0.5 ± 2.0 m/sec)

  Adelta: These are medium (2 ± 6 mm), myelinated and of intermediate velocity (12 ± 30 m/sec).

  Abeta: Large (> 10 mm), myelinated and fast (30 ± 100 m/sec)

  Under normal circumstances, only C and Adelta (but not Abeta) fibers transmit nociceptive information.

11. What type of pain sensations is transmitted by these fibers?

Ans: Upon exposure of the skin to a noxious stimulus, myelinated Adelta fibers elicit a rapid, first phase of pain, which is 'sharp' in nature. On the other hand, unmyelinated C fibers evoke a second wave of 'dull' pain.

12. What is the role of Abeta fibers in pain transmission?

Ans: In normal conditions, Abeta fibers transmit sensations related to touch, vibration, pressure and other modes of non-noxious, low intensity mechanical stimuli. However, during neuropathic pain, these fibers play an important role in transmitting pain sensations to non-noxious stimuli, i.e. allodynia.

13. What kind of analgesics can be evaluated in hot plate and tail flick tests?

Ans: Opioid analgesics prolong the jumping, licking and tail withdrawal latency in hot plate and tail flick tests. Aspirin (i.e. non-opioid) type of analgesics do not generally affect these response latencies. Therefore, these tests are used to evaluate only centrally acting analgesics including opioids (not NSAIDS including aspirin).

14. What is the advantage of tail immersion/flick tests over the hot plate test?

Ans: In contrast to hot plate procedure, the tail immersion/ flick tests can be used for repeated nociceptive evaluation using the same animal because tail withdrawal latency is not significantly affected by repeated exposure of the same animal to the testing procedure.

15. Which latency is measured in hot plate test more preferably?

Ans: The jump latency is preferred because it gives consistent and reproducible results.

16. Can the latency measurement be repeated in hot plate test and why?

Ans: The repeated latency measurements on the same animal are known to interfere with results since the animals learn to jump early, when repeatedly exposed to the hot plate.

17. What is the limitation of hot plate method?

Ans: The method has a drawback that sedatives, muscle relaxant and psychomimetics tend to give false positive tests. It means animal fail to lift the paw in the presence of these drugs and delayed paw withdrawal may be falsely assumed as an analgesic response.

18. What is the limitation of paw withdrawal threshold methods for evaluating the analgesic activities?

Ans: The paw withdrawal or tail withdrawal methods are basically the 'reflex based methods'. Some scientists document that 'reflex' measures of pain in animals are intrinsically flawed and are neither sensitive nor specific predictors of drug efficacy in man. It is stated that in these methods, motor neuron response is tested and these do not indicate pain. Furthermore, the rostral signalling pathways are ignored during measurement of only paw withdrawal threshold.

19. What is the utility of reflex based methods for pain assessment in the light of its limitation?

Ans: Despite the criticism of reflex based methods of pain assessment, paw/tail withdrawal methods are very useful. Clinically employed analgesics are found to effectively modulate paw/tail withdrawal latency or duration.

20. What are the alternatives to reflex based methods for pain assessment?

Ans: The operant models may be more useful. However, these introduce complexities such as motivational factors. These are more useful, if site of action of drug is supraspinal. However simple paw withdrawal threshold may be sufficient for drugs that act on periphery or dorsal root ganglia.

21. Who devised the hot plate technique for evaluation of analgesics?

Ans: The hot plate technique was originally devised by Woolfe and McDonald in 1944. The commonly used hot plates are based on the apparatus described by Eddy and Leimbach in 1953.

22. What are the pain tests that can distinguish opioids and NSAIDS?

Ans: The following tests can be useful for discriminating centrally acting morphine like analgesic and non-opiate analgesics.
   a. Hot plate test
   b. Radiant heat method
   c. Tail flick test
   d. Formalin test

23. What are the advantages of using carrageenan-induced paw edema (inflammation model)?

Ans: It is easy to produce, economical and less toxic material required to produce inflammation. The quantification of observations is easy.

24. What are the drawbacks of this method?

Ans: The major drawback is the unalleviated pain and deformity in this model.

25. What are the other agents that may be used in place of carrageenan?

Ans: The other irritants that may be used to produce paw edema include 4% formalin, egg white, sodium chloride, dextran, kaolin and mustard.

26. Why are local anesthetics used in preclinical study?

Ans: Local anesthetics are used to block the nerve supply to a limited area and are used only for minor and rapid procedures. This should be carried out under expert supervision for regional infiltration of surgical site, nerve blocks and for epidural and spinal anesthesia.

27. What are the advantages of hind paw edema method of evaluating anti-inflammatory drugs?

Ans: a. Rat paw edema test is easily and routinely performed.
  b. The degree of edema can be quantitatively assessed.

FOR POSTGRADUATES

28. What are the limitations of animal models of a disease?

Ans: The animal models of a disease state are generally retrospective, empirical test for measuring the effects of active compounds rather than the disease state *per se*. For example, a rat catalepsy model used to evaluate the potential antipsychotic drugs is in fact an *in vivo* model of dopamine receptor blockade.

29. What are the advantages and disadvantages of photocell count method?

Ans: *Advantages*
  a. It decreases the danger of introducing counting errors and bias of investigator.
  b. A whole group of mice (up to five) can be put in a photocell counter and count is the reading of a whole group. This count can be compared to count of another group's collective count.
  c. This procedure allows the evaluation of several drugs in a short period of time.
  d. The use of large number of animals allows for better and more reliable statistical evaluation of the data.
  Disadvantages
  a. The major limitation is with the activity counter itself. Due to burning or non-functional photoelectric cells, all the movements of the animals cannot be detected and is a source of error.

30. Which strain of mice is preferred in MES test?

Ans: CF-1 strain of mice is preferred because it is docile and tolerate the electric shock better than many other strains.

31. What is the effect of food and water on MES test?

Ans: Animals should be allowed to free access to water and food except during the actual test. Because fasting increases the severity of MES, i.e. shortens tonic flexion and prolongs tonic extension.

32. Name the scientists who paved the way of use of experimental model of epilepsy for screening of drugs.

Ans: Putnam and Merritt in 1937 demonstrated the effectiveness of anti-epileptics in electric shock seizures in laboratory animals.

33. Name the scientists who designed the electric shock machine.

Ans: Woodbury and Davenport developed electric shock seizure apparatus in 1952.

34. Which sex of mice is preferred for MES test?

Ans: Male albino mice are preferred instead of females to avoid the effect of periodic alterations of hormones (in females) on brain excitability.

35. What is the basic principle behind strychnine induced convulsions?

Ans: Glycine is an important inhibitory transmitter in motor neurons and interneurons in the spinal cord. Strychnine acts as a selective, competitive antagonist to block the inhibitory effects of glycine. The inhibition of inhibitory neurotransmitter is followed by CNS excitation. The convulsing action of strychnine is due to interference with postsynaptic inhibitory actions of glycine.

36. What is the basic principle behind picrotoxin induced convulsions?

Ans: Picrotoxin is regarded as a $GABA_A$-antagonist. GABA is the principal inhibitory neurotransmitter, which attenuates the seizure by binding to the GABA receptor and increasing the Cl^- conductance. Picrotoxin inhibits the inhibitory function of the chloride ion channel of the $GABA_A$ receptor complex to produce CNS excitation and seizures.

37. What is the basic principle behind isoniazid induced convulsions?

Ans: Isoniazid is a GABA-synthesis inhibitor. Isoniazid inhibits the synthesis of GABA to produce clonic-tonic seizures, which are antagonized by anxiolytic drugs.

38. What are tonic extensor and clonic convulsions?

Ans: The episodes of repetitive muscle spasms that persist for at least 5 seconds are called clonic convulsions. Tonic extensor convulsions are characterized by the rigid extension of the hind limbs that exceeds a 90° angle with the body.

39. What type of convulsions are produced by pentylene tetrazole (PTZ) in mice?

Ans: PTZ induces clonic convulsions at low doses (85 mg/kg s.c.); while it induces both tonic and clonic convulsions at higher doses (125 mg/kg s.c.).

40. What kind of substances/drugs can be screened by pentylenetetrazole clonic convulsions?

Ans: The drugs effective in 'absence seizures' are generally evaluated using this model. These drugs effectively inhibit the clonic convulsions.

41. What do you understand by kindling?

Ans: It is a process in which due to repeated exposures of brain to small electric shocks, there is an increased possibility for spontaneous seizure-like electrical events to occur.

In other words, it is a process in which repeated intermittent exposure of brain to a sub-threshold electrical/chemical stimulus induces electrophysiological changes so that there is permanent decrease in the threshold of excitability. Due to decreased threshold for neuronal excitability, these animals show spontaneous development of epilepsy.

42. What is the brain area involved in development of kindling?

Ans: Kindling starts in the limbic brain where it progresses from the amygdala to other side of the brain including the hippocampus, the occipital cortex, and finally to the frontal cortex.

43. What is the importance of kindling in experimental animals?

Ans: Kindling is involved in generating epilepsy in humans. During kindling, neuronal circuits are facilitated and play a key role in generating seizures in human beings.

Therefore, kindling-based epileptic models are more clinically relevant as compared to other models such as PTZ and MES.

44. What are the different methods to induce status epilepticus (SE) in rodents?

Ans: Status epilepticus (SE) may be induced in rodents by chemical agents or by electrical stimulation of brain structures. Electrical stimulation includes perforant path and self-sustaining stimulation models. Pharmacological models include kainic acid, pilocarpine, fluorothyl, organophosphates and other convulsants that induce SE in rodents.

a. *Perforant path*: In this model, anesthetized rats receive intermittent, unilateral perforant path stimulation for 24 hours. Repetitive tetanic stimulation of hippocampal afferents (perforant path) has been shown to induce SE.

b. *Self-sustaining stimulation (SSL)*: In the SSL model, a standardized amount of electrical stimulation is continuously delivered to the hippocampus to induce SE.

c. *Kainic acid (KA)*: In rats, intracerebroventricular (0.4–0.8 µg) or systemic administration (8–12 mg/kg, s.c. or i.p.) and in mice, 20–40 mg/kg, i.p. of KA induces convulsions that progress to develop SE. In these, epileptiform discharges originate in the limbic structures and propagate to other brain areas.

d. *Pilocarpine*: Systemic administration of pilocarpine (a muscarinic receptor agonist) to rats (400 mg/kg) and mice (300–350 mg/kg) induces vigorous limbic seizures that over a period of time (1–2 hours) progressively develop into limbic SE.

e. *Lithium-pilocarpine combination model*: A high dose of pilocarpine alone (400 mg/kg i.p. or s.c.) is not sufficient to induce consistent SE. Therefore, lithium is co-administered with low dose pilocarpine (20–30 mg/kg) to induce consistent SE. In order to enhance the action of pilocarpine, a small amount of lithium chloride (LiCl; 3 mEq/kg, i.p.) is given to rats prior (19 to 24 hours) to pilocarpine administration.

f. *Organophosphate pesticide model*: Systemic administration of diisopropylfluorophosphate (DFP) induces
persistent seizures and SE in rats. In this procedure,
animals are administered pyridostigmine bromide
(0.026 mg/kg, i.m.) before DFP injection and
pralidoxime chloride (2-PAM, 25 mg/kg, i.m.) along
with atropine (2 mg/kg, i.p.) after DFP injection
(1–4 mg/kg, s.c.).

g. *Fluorothyl model*: In this model, continued inhalation
of fluorothyl in a closed chamber (with constant
delivery rate of 40 ml/minute) is used to induce
prolonged seizures in animals.

**45. What are the different models to produce neuropathic
pain in rodents?**

Ans: Neuropathic pain may be produced in animals by
ligating or cutting the sciatic nerve or its different
branches. The different models of neuropathic pain
include chronic constriction injury, sciatic nerve
transection (axotomy), tibial sural nerve transection
models, etc. Neuropathic pain may also be produced by
administering some anticancer agents including
vincristine, paclitaxel and cisplatin as these drugs also
produce toxicity to nerves.

**46. What types of responses are noted down in experimental
analyses of pain?**

Ans: The somatomotor responses are noted in experiments
related to pain that vary from experiment to experiment.
These may include measurement of tail flick (mono-
synaptic reflex) in tail flick or tail immersion tests. On
the other hand, the responses such as licking/jumping
(polysynaptic reflex) are noted in case with hot plate
method that requires high degree of sensory motor co-
ordination.

47. What are the animal models of neuropathic pain?

Ans: a. Chronic constriction injury model in rat/mice
b. Partial sciatic nerve ligation model
c. Spinal nerve ligation
d. Sciatic nerve ligation
e. Tibial sural nerve transection

48. What are the behavioral tests performed to assess neuropathic pain?

Ans: a. Cold allodynia by acetone drop test

b. Mechanical hyperalgesia by pin prick and Randall-Sellito paw pressure test

c. Heat hyperalgesia by Hargreaves's paw flick test and hot plate test

49. What is the effect of age on tail flick response?

Ans: With the increase in the age of the rodents, the keratinization on the tail produces heat insulating effect and decreases the flick response to heat.

50. Which part of the tail is more sensitive to heat stimuli?

Ans: The distal part is more sensitive compared to proximal part of tail.

51. What do you understand by % MPE?

Ans: It stands for maximal possible effect and it is used to calculate the analgesic effect of drugs in tail flick and hot plate method. Its formula is

$$\%MPE = \frac{[\text{Post-drug latency}] - [\text{Pre-drug latency}]}{[\text{Cut-off time}] - [\text{Pre-drug latency}]} \times 100$$

52. What are the limitations of hind paw edema method used for evaluating anti-inflammatory drugs?

Ans: a. The subcutaneous tissue of hind paw has significant content of 5-HT. Therefore, 5-HT antagonist may also reduce edema even if these do not possess significant anti-inflammatory activity, e.g. bromolysergic acid and diethylamide tartarate.

b. Mechanistically, this model only represents the acute vascular response to injury (concerned with edema). It is not representative of WBC events that are crucial part of inflammation.

Based on this, it may be summarized that suppression of rat hind paw does not seem to give a particularly valid assessment of clinical anti-inflammatory drugs in current use.

53. **What are the drugs that are effectively evaluated using ultraviolet erythema method?**

Ans: There is a strong correlation between suppression of ultraviolet induced erythema in Guinea pigs and clinical efficacy in rheumatoid arthritis.

The reason for the correlation does not seem obvious because ultraviolet erythema depends on dilation of arterioles (early and transient reaction of inflammation). On the other hand, clinical efficacy of anti-rheumatic drugs depends on suppression of cellular exudation and proliferation.

54. **Name the instrument used to record mean arterial blood pressure in rats and other animals.**

Ans: Candon's blood pressure manometer.

55. **How does Candon's blood pressure manometer differs from conventional manometer?**

Ans: Candon's blood pressure manometer is specially designed manometer in which the main limb of the manometer is a long narrow tube (28 cm long and 2.5 mm in diameter), and its other limb is replaced by a wider reservoir of 2.5 cm diameter. The result is that even with a small fall in the mercury level, there is a significant rise in the mercury level in a small bore of limb. Therefore, the sensitivity of this monometer is twice than as compared to the normal U-shaped manometer (Fig. 5.1).

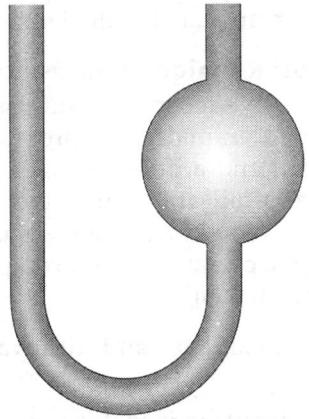

Fig. 5.1: Schematic diagram of Candon's blood pressure manometer

56. What are the different methods of determining blood pressure in animals?

Ans: The blood pressure is determined in animals by direct (invasive, surgical method) or by indirect (non-invasive) methods (by a tail cuff technique).

57. How is blood pressure measured by direct or invasive method? What is its major limitation?

Ans: In this method, the animal is anesthetized, carotid artery is cannulated and connected to blood pressure transducer to note mean arterial blood pressure.

The major limitation is that, the blood pressure cannot be measured over a period of time by this technique. In other words, repeated measurement of blood pressure over an extended period of time is not possible because the animal cannot be kept in surgical position for extended period.

58. What is the principle of tail cuff technique of blood pressure measurement?

Ans: The principle of determining blood pressure by tail cuff method is analogous to sphygmomanometry in humans. In this method (indirect tail cuff method), the systolic blood pressure is measured by inflating the cuff above the suspected systolic blood pressure (at this pressure pulse will be diminished). Thereafter, the pressure in cuff is slowly released and as pressure falls below systolic blood pressure, the pulse reappears. The pressure at which pulse reappears is called systolic blood pressure.

59. What is tail cuff technique of measuring blood pressure?

Ans: It is non-invasive technique and uses un-anesthetized, but restrained animals. The procedure uses a special inflatable cuff and a pulse detector and both are fitted over the rat's tail and connected to blood pressure recorder. The blood pressure measurement is based on monitoring the pulsatile blood flow (pulses) in the caudal artery in the rat's tail.

60. What are the advantages and disadvantages of tail cuff technique?

Ans: The major advantage is that it is non-invasive and easy to perform. Unlike in surgical method, the blood pressure can be measured over an extended period of time. Therefore, multiple readings from a same animal may be taken on different days. The disadvantage include that it only measures systolic blood pressure. There are a lot of variations in blood pressure reading due to multiple reasons including movement of animal in restrainer.

61. What are the chemicals used to induce the hypertension in rats?

Ans: Deoxycorticosterone acetate (DOCA)-salt is mainly used to induce hypertension in rats. This is based on the theory that mineralocorticoid has sodium retaining properties, which increases the plasma and extracellular volume. The increase in plasma volume is associated with rise in blood pressure. The hypertensive effect is increased by salt loading and unilateral nephrectomy in rats.

62. What type of hypertension may be induced by surgical methods in animals?

Ans: By surgical method, renal hypertension (acute and chronic) and neurogenic hypertension can be induced in experimental animals.

63. What is neurogenic hypertension and how is it induced in dogs?

Ans: Neurogenic hypertension is due to excessive activation of the sympathetic nervous system. In this method, both the carotid arteries are cleared up to the bifurcation of the internal and external carotid arteries. The carotid sinus nerves are isolated, ligated and sectioned and a bilateral vagotomy is performed to produce neurogenic hypertension (mean arterial pressure more than 150 mm Hg).

64. What do you mean by renal hypertension?

Ans: The ischemia of the kidney elevates the blood pressure by activating the renin-angiotensin system and resulting high blood pressure is termed renal hypertension. Experimentally, both acute and chronic renal hypertensions may be induced in rats.

65. How can acute renal hypertension be induced in rats?

Ans: In rats, acute renal hypertension can be induced by clamping the left renal artery for 4 hours. After reopening of artery vessel, accumulated renin is released into circulation. The protease renin catalyzes the formation of angiotensin II which leads to acute hypertension.

66. **How can chronic renal hypertension be induced in rats?**

Ans: Chronic hypertension may be induced by clamping renal arteries, i.e. one-kidney-one-clip (1K1C), two-kidney-one-clip (2K1C) methods in rats and by wrapping method in dogs.

67. **What are the one-kidney-one-clip (1K1C) and two-kidney-one-clip (2K1C) methods?**

Ans: In the 2K1C model, one renal artery is constricted to chronically reduce renal perfusion, and the other kidney remains untouched. In the 1K1C model, one kidney is removed, and the other undergoes artery constriction. In both models, the earliest phase of hypertension is characterized by a rapid rise in plasma renin in response to low renal arterial pressure and by the consequent increase in circulating Ang. II.

68. **What are different strains of genetic hypertension in rats?**

Ans: Genetically hypertensive (GH) rats are "spontaneously hypertensive rats (Akamoto-Aoki)" = (SHR) or "Wistar-Kyoto rats" = (WKY), Milan hypertensive strain" = (MHS), Spontaneously hypertensive stroke-prone strain = (SHRSP).

69. **What is Milan hypertensive strain (MHS)?**

Ans: This hypertensive strain is derived from Wistar rats by brother–sister mating by the group of Bianchi et al (1974, 1986) at the University of Milan. These rats show a cell membrane defect resulting in abnormal kidney function and hypertension.

70. **What is spontaneously hypertensive stroke-prone strain (SHRSP)?**

Ans: SHRSP rats have an increased sympathetic tone and hypertension. These are characterized by hemorrhagic lesions of the brain with motor disturbances followed by death.

71. What are chemical methods to induce myocardial infarction?

Ans: Injection of natural as well as synthetic sympathomimetic agents in high dose results in cardiac necrosis. Administration of 5.25 and 8.5 mg/kg isoproterenol s.c. on two consecutive days produces infarct like myocardiac lesions in rats.

72. What is surgical method to induce myocardial infarction?

Ans: Occlusion of coronary artery in anesthetized dogs/rats can induce infarction.

73. Why is LAD occluded for studying ischemic effects on rat heart?

Ans: LAD is left anterior descending coronary artery that supplies the largest part of heart, i.e. left ventricles. Therefore, the occlusion of LAD is preferred for producing local ischemia in rats.

74. What are different arrythmogenic stimuli to induce arrhythmia?

Ans: Arrythmogenic stimuli can be divided into three groups: Chemical, electrical and mechanical.

75. Describe chemically-induced arrhythmia.

Ans: Administration of anesthetics like chloroform, ether, halothane (sensitizing agents) followed by a precipitating stimulus such as intravenous adrenaline, or cardiac glycosides (usually ouabain), aconitine, and veratrum alkaloids cause arrhythmias. The sensitivity to these arrhythmogenic substances differs among various species.

76. Describe electrically induced arrhythmias.

Ans: The possibilities to produce arrhythmias by electrical stimulation of the heart and the difficulties for evaluation of anti-arrhythmic drugs by this approach have been discussed by Szekeres (1971). Serial electrical stimulation result in flutter and fibrillation and arrhythmia can be induced with features common to main types of arrhythmias of clinical importance.

77. Describe mechanically induced arrhythmias.

Ans: Arrhythmias can be induced directly by ischemia or by reperfusion. After ischemia either by infarction or by coronary ligation, several phases of arrhythmias are induced. The two stage coronary artery ligation technique described by Harris (1950) produces late arrhythmias.

78. Describe aconitine induced arrhythmia in rats.

Ans: Alkaloid aconitine persistently activates sodium channels. Infusion of aconitine 5 µg/kg dissolved in 0.1 N HNO_3 into sephaneous vein induces ventricular arrhythmia in rats.

79. Why is mongolian gerbil preferred in model of stroke and multi-infarct cerebral dysfunction?

Ans: The mongolian gerbil (*Meriones unguiculatus*) is extremely susceptible to cerebral ischemia due to carotid occlusion because of the peculiar anatomy. There is occurrence of an incomplete circle of Willis without posterior communicating artery and a frequently rudimentary anterior communicating artery. Clamping of both carotid arteries induces a bilateral temporary brain ischemia. The gerbil is known to develop selective neuronal damage in the CA1 sector of the hippocampus following brief periods of forebrain ischemia.

80. What are the different methods to induce cerebral ischemia?

Ans: The different methods include middle cerebral artery occlusion in rats (MCA), carotid artery occlusion, and photochemically induced focal cerebral ischemia.

81. What is fluvography?

Ans: It is a cerebral blood flow measuring device consisting of thermo probe which is attached to the tissue to record the heat transport continuously. The device depends on having an electrically heated part and an unheated reference point. The difference in temperature between these points is a function of local blood flow. An increase in flow tends to lower the local temperature by carrying away the heat gain and vice versa.

82. What is laser Doppler effect?

Ans: The principle of laser effect is based on the fact that a laser light beam directed on tissue is scattered by static structure as well as by moving cells. Light beam scattered by moving red cells undergo a frequency shift according to the Doppler effect, while beams scattered in static tissue alone remain unshifted in frequency. The number of Doppler shifts per time is recorded as a measure for erythrocyte flow in a given volume.

83. Where is laser Doppler effect used?

Ans: Laser Doppler effect determines relative changes in microcirculatory blood flow. Therefore, it is used to detect test compounds that improve blood supply of the brain or the flow of red blood cells in the ischemic skeletal muscles.

84. What is thromboelastography?

Ans: It is a device that provides a continuous recording of the process of blood coagulation and subsequent clot retraction. It is used to evaluate drugs affecting the fibrinolytic compounds.

85. What is radio telemetry?

Ans: Radio telemetry allows the recording of cardiovascular parameters in conscious, free moving animals.

86. What is the chemical method of inducing type II diabetes in animals?

Ans: A single low dose streptozotocin (40–45 mg/kg in young adult rats and 20–30 mg/kg in older rats) produces NIDDM. Otherwise, a dose of 65 mg/kg in rats and 200 mg/kg in mice produces full blown IDDM.

Alternatively, streptozotocin may be injected i.p. or i.v. in neonates within two days of birth to result in NIDDM in later life. Neonatal injection of streptozotocin quickly destroys most of the beta cells which is followed by gradual regeneration of about half of the population.

87. What is the major limitation of streptozotocin or alloxan models of IDDM?

Ans: The immediate high mortality rate associated with these models is the major limitation.

88. How can it be overcome?

Ans: The high mortality due to streptozotocin injection is due to very high levels of insulin in the blood due to massive destruction of beta cells. A very high level of insulin produces hypoglycemia which is fatal in nature. It can be overcome by adding sucrose in the drinking water for 2–3 days after streptozotocin injection.

89. What are the different animal models of schizophrenia?

Ans: a. Amphetamine-induced hyperactivity
b. Amphetamine-induced stereotypy
c. Phencyclidine disruption of prepulse
d. Inhibition of startle in rats

90. What are the common animal models of affective illness (depression)?

Ans: a. Behavioral despair test in rat
b. Forced swimming test in mouse
c. Tail suspension test in mouse

91. What are the common animal models of anxiety?

Ans: a. Elevated plus maze test in rats/mice
b. Ultrasonic vocalization of isolated rats pups

92. What are the animal models of benign prostatic hyperplasia?

Ans: a. Rise in prostate pressure and blood pressure in anesthetized dogs in response to phenylephrine.
b. Rise in prostate pressure and blood pressure in anesthetized dogs in response to hypogastric nerve stimulation and phenylephrine administration.

93. What are the animals preferred for testing antiemetics agents?

Ans: Cats or dogs are generally employed. Rodents cannot be used because they lack vomiting center in the brain.

94. What are the preferable animals for studying fibrinolytic system?

Ans: The fibrinolytic system in rabbit is qualitatively same as that in human plasma. Therefore, the results obtained in rabbits reflect the effects of drugs in man.

95. What is the limitation of rat as an animal for evaluating diuretics?

Ans: Diuretics are evaluated on rats including benzthiadiazines. However, some diuretics do not produce diuresis in rats though they are known to produce diuresis in man and other species, e.g. mercurial. So there is a possibility of overlooking a diuretic if rat is the only species being evaluated. Accordingly it is desirable to test at least two species for evaluating diuretics.

96. What do you understand by spatial learning?

Ans: In this test, rat uses spatial information provided by distal cues in the room to locate the target.

97. What are the memory evaluation tests based on spatial memory?

Ans: Morris water maze test and radial arm maze test

98. What are the advantages of Morris water maze test over radial arm maze test?

Ans: The advantages of Morris water maze test over radial arm maze include:

   a. Animals are trained in shorter period (1 week), on Morris water maze while radial arm maze studies require several weeks of training.

   b. Intramaze cues like odor are eliminated in water pool

   c. The motor movement related problems can be detected in trial period.

   d. The animals are not deprived from food during the test.

   e. Water maze is aversively motivated while arm maze is appetitive motivated.

99. What are the disadvantages of Morris water maze test?

Ans: The disadvantages of Morris water maze test include:

   a. Water immersion itself may cause endocrinological or other stress effects, which may interfere with drug testing.

   b. Experiment must be run by hand rather than automated equipment.

100. What is the most important limitation of radial arm maze test?

Ans: This test is appetitively motivated task. Therefore, the drugs that inhibit the appetite (anorectic agent) impair the learning in this test. Furthermore, the hypothalamic lesions also affect appetite, and therefore, affect learning in this test.

101. What do you mean by delayed matching test (DMT)?

Ans: Delayed matching test assesses the type of memory often impaired by brain damage in humans. In this test, the animals are asked to compare its short term memory of a visual stimulus with an actual stimulus. At the beginning of the trial, one or more stimuli are presented as the sample. After a short delay, during which the sample stimulus is removed, the animal is given a choice between two or more visual stimuli, one of which is the same as the sample. The animal must remember the object (stimulus) that was shown first. DMT assesses the animal's ability to remember information about the first object during the delay.

102. What is the practical example of delayed matching test?

Ans: A rat is placed in a start box from which it could see three light bulbs, one of which is lit to signal the presence of food in the corresponding arm of the maze. After the light is turned off, the rat is kept in the start box for a period of time and then released. In order to get the food, the rat has to "remember" which of the lights has been on. Rat could perform the task successfully with a delay of up to 10 seconds.

103. What are the advantages of delayed matching test?

Ans: a. The test has high face validity because humans require this type of memory everyday. Require this type of memory everyday.

b. The delayed matching test and other models that employ choice procedures are particularly useful in separating memory from performance.

104. Why are rodents preferred for spatial memory related tests?

Ans: The ecology of rodents makes these animals very efficient in spatial discrimination learning within a few trials. The rodents master the spatial learning within a few days. The errors encountered during locating the targets are not solely due to their inability to remember the correct solution, but their tendency to explore alternative pathway.

105. What is passive avoidance?

Ans: It is used to describe the experiments in which animals learn to avoid noxious events by suppressing a particular behavior. It is also described as "inhibitory avoidance".

106. What are the different memory tests based on the principle of passive avoidance?

Ans: These include:
   a. Step down
   b. Step through
   c. Two compartment test
   d. Up-hill avoidance test

107. What is active avoidance?

Ans: Active avoidance learning is a fundamental behavioral phenomenon. The animals learn to control the administration of unconditioned stimulus by appropriate reaction to conditioned stimulus preceding the noxious stimulus.

108. What are the different memory tests based on active avoidance behavior?

Ans: Runaway avoidance, shuttle box avoidance and jumping avoidance.

Experimental Design, Bioassay and Toxicity Studies

6

FOR UNDERGRADUATES AND POSTGRADUATES

1. What is the use of control/normal/negative control group?

Ans: This group is used to assess the impact of external variables (environmental) or other possible unwanted factors other than the test drug on the biological response.

2. What is the role of vehicle control group?

Ans: These groups assess whether vehicle alone produces significant biological effect or not. It is given in the same schedule as that of drug treatment and the effects of this group are compared with the control/normal group.

3. What is the relevance of sham control group?

Ans: Sham control group is employed to assess any significant effect of surgical procedure or other special treatment technique such as ICV injection in the animals. The response of this group is compared with the control/ normal group or vehicle control group.

4. What are positive control groups?

Ans: These are the groups in which a standard drug with a known biological effect is administered. Therefore, in these groups, a biological effect is expected.

Sometimes, these may be a disease model group in which definite pathological changes are observed due to treatment with chemicals or bacteria.

This group is included to ascertain the accuracy of methodology employed in experimentation. The failure to obtain a biological response with a standard drug or failure to induce a disease with known chemical/bacteria denotes the inaccuracy of procedure.

5. **What do you understand by comparative control groups?**

Ans: In comparative control groups, a direct comparison is made between the biological effect of a test drug and that of a standard drug (effective first line drug).

6. **What do you understand by reproducibility?**

Ans: Reproducibility means repetitiveness. In other words, it means that results obtained in laboratory can be reproduced using the same process, method and material in a distinct laboratory under different conditions, different apparatus and different temperatures.

7. **What do you understand by latin square design?**

Ans: Latin square design is an experimental design that can be used to control the random variation of two factors. The design is arranged with an equal number of rows and columns, so that all combinations of possible values for the two variables can be tested multiple times. This design is used to reduce the effect of random factors.

8. **Give example of latin square for four doses.**

Ans: For four dose schedule, different types of latin square may be designed. It should be noted that in any row, the same dose is not repeated.

For example:

```
A B C D      A B C D
B A D C      B A D C
C D A B      C D A B
D C B A      D C A B
```

9. **Why is it necessary to add doses in latin square design in bioassay?**

Ans: The sensitivity of tissue varies with time during the course of experimentation. Furthermore, the response of a dose is affected by the size of previous dose. Therefore, it is necessary that doses should be evenly distributed throughout the assay. Furthermore, it is also necessary to add doses in a random manner, which is possible by using latin square design.

10. What is validity?

Ans: Validity refers to how well a test measures what it is supposed to measure.

11. What do you mean by face validity?

Ans: This term is very commonly used to describe the rationality of animal model. Face validity refers to the similarity of symptoms produced in the disease model and the naturally occurring disease in humans. It means how closely an animal model resembles the human disease.

In other words, it is defined as 'the degree of phenomenological similarity between the animal model and the specific symptoms of the human disease'. For example, a new drug was to produce an abnormal posture in rats called catatonia and tests on human might show it to be an antipsychotic. These tests have low face validity.

12. What is predictive validity?

Ans: Predictive validity is often used in preclinical testing and is used to describe the ability of animal model to identify drugs with potential therapeutic value in humans. In other words, it is used to describe whether the drugs effective in ameliorating the disease in an animal model are effective in attenuating human disease. It is used to correlate the potency in the animal model with clinical potency.

13. What is construct validity?

Ans: A model is said to have high construct validity, if response obtained in that model is very close to that observed in clinical setting. Furthermore, from the response of model, the response in clinical setup can be predicted.

In other words, if the drug effects in the clinical laboratory test closely parallel or predict the clinical effect, the measures may be said to demonstrate construct/empirical validity.

14. What is random error?

Ans: This type of error is unbiased and is usually on either side of mean. The observed values vary randomly from the true value, some being larger and some smaller. These are commonly related to imprecision of measurement done by the experimenter. These may also be due to unknown and unpredictable changes in the experiment. These changes may occur due to measuring instruments or in the environmental conditions.

15. What is systematic error?

Ans: Systematic error is biased and is usually on one side of mean. Systematic error occurs due to inaccurate or uncalibrated instruments, e.g. BP apparatus, weighing balance. Uncalibrated instruments will give either a high or lower values as compared to true values, but these values will be always one sided. This type of error can be avoided by recalibration of instrument.

16. Define reliability.

Ans: Reliability is the degree to which an assessment tool produces consistent and reproducible results. A method or procedure is said to have high reliability, if results obtained under defined conditions of testing may be reproduced, when repeated time to time in that laboratory and from one laboratory to another.

17. Differentiate validity and reliability.

Ans: Reliability means consistency of a measurement and it may be determined by performing tests. The consistency in results denotes high reliability. It means a method of measurement or procedure for testing is reliable and consistent results can be produced on repetition of experiments in one laboratory and to another laboratory.

The test which is employed for measuring a parameter (say CNS stimulant activity) may have validity only if a test employed to measure the parameter is actually measuring what it is supposed to measure. A test may have good consistency, but may lack the validity, if the test is not actually measuring what is supposed to measure. It is difficult to measure and is determined by internal validity, construct validity, and external validity.

18. What is the crossover design?

Ans: In a crossover design, same individual is assigned to receive two or more treatments in a particular sequence. An individual in a crossover study receives the drug treatment (or placebo) in the first period. Thereafter, after a suitably long washout period, the same individual receives placebo (or drug treatment).

19. What are the advantages of the crossover design?

Ans: The greatest advantages of the crossover design are:

a. Individuals act as their own controls. Therefore, the inter-individual variability is reduced.

b. Lesser number of individuals may be required in a trial.

20. What are the disadvantages of the crossover design?

Ans: a. In crossover designs, it may be difficult to interpret the results. As all individuals receive more than one treatment, there can be a carryover effect of one treatment (from early periods) to another treatment (during subsequent periods) leading to a biased effects.

b. These are not applicable to all therapeutic indications. Crossover trials are ideally suited for chronic indications that do not vary in severity over time including hypercholesterolemia or hypertension. For acute conditions (including pain) that got treated, crossover design cannot be applied.

21. What are concurrently controlled, parallel group design studies?

Ans: In parallel group trial, individuals are randomly assigned to two or more distinct treatment groups. The two parallel groups, one group is termed 'drug treatment group' and other is termed the 'placebo treatment group'. The latter functions as the control group, so it is termed concurrently controlled, parallel group design studies.

Sometimes this design is also called 'placebo-controlled parallel group design', because the control employed is a placebo.

22. What does the word concurrently implies in concurrently controlled, parallel group design studies?

Ans: The term "concurrently" refers to the fact that the individuals in the 'placebo treatment group' are participating in the trial at the same time as those in the 'drug treatment group'.

23. What is the difference between a clinical endpoint and a surrogate endpoint?

Ans: Surrogate endpoints are biomarkers that substitute for the clinical endpoint by predicting its likely behavior.

24. What are double blind studies?

Ans: In double blind studies, both investigator and patients are unaware of the type of treatment a patient is receiving, i.e. whether a patient is receiving an active drug or a placebo.

25. What is the difference between pragmatic studies and explanatory studies?

Ans: *Explanatory studies (efficacy)*: These studies are done under 'ideal' or 'laboratory' conditions. It allows tight control over patient selection, treatment and follow up. These studies provide insight into biological mechanisms. However, these studies are not generalizable to clinical practice.

Pragmatic studies (effectiveness): These studies are used for 'decision making'. These are conducted under 'normal' conditions that reflect the circumstances under which the medical care is provided.

26. What do you understand by bioassay?

Ans: Bioassay is defined as the estimation of potency of an active principle in a unit quantity of preparation or detection and measurement of the concentration of the substance in a preparation using biological material including living tissues, microorganisms, immune cells or animals.

27. What is the importance of bioassay?

Ans: Bioassay is the only method of assay if:

a. Active principle of drug is unknown or cannot be isolated, e.g. insulin, posterior pituitary extract, etc.

b. Chemical method is either not available or if available it is too complex and insensitive or requires higher dose, e.g. insulin, acetylcholine, etc.

c. Chemical composition is not known, e.g. long-acting thyroid stimulants.

d. Chemical composition of drug is different, but have the same pharmacological actions and vice versa, e.g. cardiac glycosides, catecholamines, etc.

28. What is the principle of bioassay?

Ans: The basic principle of bioassay is to compare the biological effects of a test substance with the international standard preparation of the same compound. Thereafter, it is determined how much test substance is required to produce the same effect as produced by the standard.

29. What are disadvantages of bioassay?

Ans: • Quantitative accuracy falls below that is obtainable from chemical analysis

• It is less sensitive method as compared to chemical assays

• The techniques and interpretation involved often vary from laboratory to laboratory

• Less precise, time-consuming and more expensive to conduct

30. Classify different types of bioassay.

Ans:

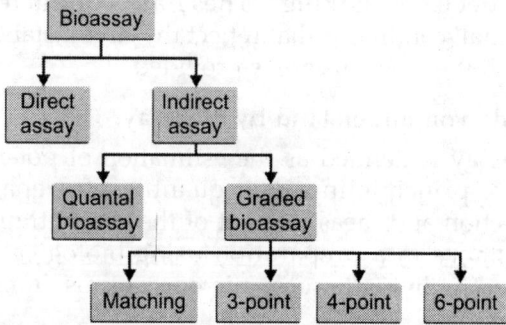

31. What do you mean by direct bioassay?

Ans: In direct bioassay, the response produced by test drug is compared with standard drug. The doses where responses produced are equivalent and determined, and from that potency of test drug is calculated. For example, decrease in BP caused by two drugs is compared, when decrease in BP is same, then the two doses are said to be equivalent. In this type of assay, biological variation is not taken into account and reproducibility is not good. Therefore, it is less accurate method. However, it is less time-consuming method.

32. What do you mean by quantal bioassay?

Ans: It is a method in which effect produced is all or none, i.e. either a response will be produced or not, e.g. the potency of digitalis preparation is noted by quantal bioassay in which response is either death or survival (all-or-none) of dog or cat.

33. What do you mean by graded bioassay?

Ans: In this case, there is gradual change in response with change of dose of a drug and a dose-response phenomenon is observed. In other words, as the dose is varied, there is variation in response. There are different methods of doing graded bioassay including matching bioassay, bracketing assay, interpolation method and multiple point bioassays (three-point bioassay, four-point bioassay and six-point bioassay).

34. What do you mean by matching bioassay?

Ans: In this case, test and standard are matched by trial and error process until they produce equal effects. It is employed for small sample size.

Its major advantage is that there is no need to plot dose-response curve. It is less time consuming and therefore, it is useful, if sensitivity of preparation is not stable.

However, there are number of disadvantages that include: Match is purely subjective; experimental error cannot be determined; it does not give idea of dose-response relationship.

35. What is bracketing method of bioassay?

Ans: The response of test compound is bracketed between two responses (greater and smaller) of standard substance. The strength of an unknown compound is determined by simple interpolation of this bracketed response on the dose axis. It is used when test sample is too small. However, the precision and reliability of this method is poor.

36. What are the major advantages and disadvantages of matching and bracketing methods?

Ans: The major advantages and disadvantages of matching and bracketing methods are as follows:

Advantages
- Faster
- Can be completed when amount of test drug available is small
- Does not involve complicated calculations

Disadvantages
- Match is subjective
- Exact match may not always be possible
- No evidence of parallelism/discrimination
- Does not permit calculation of variation.

37. What do you mean by 3-point, 4-point and 6-point bioassays?

Ans: These bioassays are based on the assumption of the dose-response relationship. Log dose-response curve is plotted and the dose of test producing the same response as produced by standard is directly read from graph.

In **3-point** bioassay, 2 doses of the standard and 1 dose of the test are used.

In **4-point** bioassay, 2 doses of the standard and 2 doses of test are used.

In **6-point** bioassay, 3 doses of the standard and 3 doses of test are used.

38. When a 3-point bioassay is employed?

Ans: It is used when test solution is in short supply and when a high degree of accuracy is not necessary.

39. How do the doses calculated in 4-point bioassay?

Ans: First of all, DRC of standard is plotted to note down the dose that produce minimum and maximum response. Thereafter, the doses of 'test' and 'standard' which produce response not less than 25% of maximum response and not more than 75% of maximum response are selected. Sometimes, if tissue response is very steep with rise in dose, then it is better to choose the responses that lie between 25% and 50% of maximum. Because the tissue takes longer time to recover after contraction with higher doses.

40. What are recent applications of 6-point bioassay?

Ans: a. Microbiological assay of vit B_{12}

b. Analgesic assay of buprenorphine and morphine

c. Diazyme's cystatin-C assay: A marker of renal disease

d. Comparative assays of erythropoietin standards

41. What are the advantages of multiple point assays over matching/bracketing bioassay?

Ans: 1. In multiple point method, the doses of standard are selected on the basis of DRC, where the linear relationship is observed between dose and response (usually the middle portion of DRC). On the other hand, the selection of standard and test doses in matching/bracketing method is arbitrary and selected doses not necessarily fall in the linear region of DRC. Therefore, the selection of doses at nonlinear region of DRC reduces the sensitivity and also, the accuracy of test.

2. In multiple point method, the comparison of response of standard and test are done at different dose levels depending upon the type of test employed. For example, in 4-point bioassay, the comparison is made between two doses of test and two doses of standard. Therefore, multiple reading of test and standard are taken to obtain a single representative value to reduce the overall biological error.

3. Furthermore, order of addition of doses of test and standard is done using Latin-square design in order to avoid any discrepancy in biological response.

42. Which is the most preferred multipoint bioassay?

Ans: Four-point bioassay is most commonly employed among different types of multipoint bioassay. It provides adequate accuracy and removes bias effectively. Though 6-point bioassay is more accurate, yet it is not preferred because it is very complicated in executing the assay along with very complicated calculations.

43. What do you understand by acute toxicity study?

Ans: It is defined as the study comprising shorter duration (day 0 to 1 week).

44. What do you understand by sub-acute/sub-chronic toxicity study?

Ans: It is defined as the study comprising shorter to medium duration (> 1 week to 12 weeks).

45. What do you understand by chronic toxicity study?

Ans: It is defined as the study comprising longer duration (> 12 weeks to 24 weeks or even up to 18 months in higher animals like dog or monkeys).

46. What do you understand by therapeutic index?

Ans: The therapeutic index of a drug is usually defined as the ratio of LD_{50} to ED_{50}, which indicates how selective the drug is in eliciting its desired effect. The therapeutic index of a drug is the ratio of the dose that results in an undesired effect to that which results in a desired effect. Higher the therapeutic index, more safe is drug.

47. Define toxic dose level (TDL).

Ans: Toxic dose level (TDL) is defined as the lowest dose of a drug which does not produce any lethality, but produces pathology changes in hematological, biochemical, clinical or morphological parameters.

48. Define LD_{50}.

Ans: It is defined as the dose of a given drug which produces mortality in 50% of total treated animal, preferably in the most sensitive species model.

49. What is the effect of choices of species in teratogenic studies?

Ans: The teratogenic agents produce different actions in different species, e.g.

Thalidomide produces malformation in rabbits but is safe in rats.

Azathioprine produces teratogenic effects in rabbits but is safe in rats and mice.

Cortisone is potent teratogenic in mouse but do not produce any abnormal effect in rats.

50. What are the different animals employed for teratogenic studies with advantages and limitations?

Ans: Rats: Mostly rats are used as reference animals. Its advantages include that it has high fertility rate and very low rate of spontaneous malformation. Its major limitation is that various known teratogenic agents like thalidomide, azathiopurine do not produce malformation in rats.

Mouse: It is much more susceptible to teratogenic agent in comparison to rats. The major limitation include relatively high rate of spontaneous malformation.

Rabbit: It is a very favorable animal for teratogenic studies. However, it also develops spontaneous anomalies. Besides this, rat, mice and rabbits have short pregnancy time and easy to handle.

Guinea pigs: It has placental similarities with human and its gestational hormonal balance is closer to humans. Its major limitation is long pregnancy time (three times longer) and each litter has two fetus.

Biochemical Techniques

7

FOR UNDERGRADUATES AND POSTGRADUATES

1. What do you understand by reference value?

Ans: These are the values of a particular parameter obtained from healthy individuals. The test values are compared with reference values and conclusion is made about the state (healthy or diseased) of an individual.

2. What is an analytical method?

Ans: It is a set of instructions which describe the procedure, materials and equipment necessary to obtain a result.

3. What is calibration?

Ans: It is the process of relating the values indicated on the scale of an instrument to the quantity required to be measured.

4. What do you mean by standard?

Ans: It is the material or solution with which the sample is compared to obtain the result.

5. What are the different types of standards?

Ans: a. *Arbitrary standard*: This standard contains an unknown quantity of the specified substance. The content is assigned by convention and expressed in arbitrary units.

   Examples: International biological standard for heparin, insulin, etc.

   b. *Internal standard*: It is not normally present in the specimen and is clearly distinguishable from the substance to be analyzed. It is added in a known quantity to the sample for the purpose of correcting results for inaccuracy.

c. *Primary standard*: A substance of known chemical composition and purity is used for preparing primary standard solution. Its concentration is determined by dissolving a weighed amount of primary standard material in an appropriate solvent.

d. *Secondary standard solution*: The concentration of these solutions is determined by an analytical method using primary standard solutions.

6. What are the reliability criteria of an analytical method?

Ans: Accuracy, precision, specificity and sensitivity

7. What do you mean by sensitivity?

Ans: The ability of an analytical method to detect the smallest quantity of a component. It is mainly expressed by detection limits. The smallest quantity that may be measured by an analytical method is referred to as sensitivity of method.

8. What do you mean by specificity?

Ans: The ability of an analytical method to determine only the component that we wish to determine, without determining the other related components.

9. What is the difference between definitive method and reference method?

Ans: **Definitive method:** An analytic procedure for the measurement of a specified analyte in a specified material, which is known to give essentially the true value for the concentration of the analyte.

Reference method: An analytic procedure sufficiently free of random or systematic error to make it useful for validating proposed new analytic procedures for the same analyte.

10. How is the specificity of analytical method reduced?

Ans: The reduction of specificity of an analytical method may be due to:

a. *Interference*: Due to presence of non-reacting substances, e.g. turbidity, hemoglobin in sample, these interfering substances do not show any chemical reaction, but interferes with end point determination, e.g. color development.

b. *Non-specificity*: Due to presence of 'related material' in the sample along with the component that we wish to determine. The related material themselves show chemical reaction and compete with 'component' that is to be determined. This reduces the specificity of reaction and introduces the non-specificity. For example, presence of number of related sugars such as fructose may impart non-specificity in glucose determination.

11. How is the Precision index calculated?

Ans: The Precision index is calculated by the following formula:

Precision index = $(100 \times (X_a - X_b)/\text{true value})/\text{Coefficient}$ of variation $\times 100$ where X_a, X_b are the values obtained after repeated measurements.

The value is calculated for 10 days and average result is noted as precision index.

12. How is the accuracy index calculated?

Ans: Accuracy index = $(100 \times (X_a - \text{true value})/\text{true value})/$ Coefficient of variation $\times 100$

It is related to precision index, but in this case the observed results are compared to true value.

13. What is the most important precaution that should be taken during plasma or serum separation?

Ans: It is very important to avoid hemolysis of blood during plasma and serum separation. The presence of red coloration (indicative of hemolysis) makes the plasma unsuitable for determination.

14. What are the steps that may be taken to avoid hemolysis?

Ans: Hemolysis is avoided by decreasing the mechanical breakdown of RBC. The blood should be added in a container gently. Excessive amount of anticoagulant should be avoided. Both should be mixed gently. Centrifugation to isolate plasma should be done at slower speed.

15. What is the optimum time of clotting for isolating serum from blood?

Ans: The longer the time allowed for clotting, the more serum is obtained. The optimum time period is 15–30 minutes. However, on keeping the blood for clotting for longer period, the changes in distribution of substances between cells and serum occurs, which may influence the results.

16. What are the different anticoagulants used and write their advantages and disadvantages?

Ans: a. *Heparin*: It is the most satisfactory anticoagulant because it does not interfere or change RBC volume. However, it is more costly than other anticoagulants.

b. *EDTA*: It produces anticoagulant effect by chelating calcium ions. It also does not alter the RBC volume and hence, it is commonly used for blood collected for hematological examination.

c. *Oxalates*: Potassium oxalate acts by precipitating the calcium.

d. *Sodium citrate*: It does not precipitate calcium, but converts it into non-ionized form.

e. *Sodium fluoride*: It has to be used in larger amount than oxalates and citrates. It is mainly used as preservative because it inhibits red cell metabolism and bacterial action.

17. What are the changes that may be induced in blood on keeping for long period?

Ans: When blood is kept at room temperature for long period, various undesirable changes occurs in blood including:

a. CO_2 dissolved in plasma diffuses to air and hence, blood becomes more alkaline.

b. The glucose content decreases due to glycolysis.

c. Increase in plasma inorganic phosphate due to degradation of ATP to ADP and AMP. Therefore, plasma should be separated in short time after separation of blood.

d. Formation of ammonia from urea due to presence of bacteria. So blood should be kept sterile.

e. Passage of substances across RBC—Potassium diffuses from RBC to plasma due to concentration gradient.

18. How blood should be stored?

Ans: To avoid the undesirable changes, blood should be stored at 4 °C in a refrigerator for up to 24 hours. Otherwise, it should be stored at much lower temperature, if it is to be stored for longer period.

19. What is the reason for the choice of whole blood, serum or plasma for determination of particular component?

Ans: The choice of blood, serum or plasma actually depends upon the type of substrate that is to be measured. However, in general plasma or serum is mostly employed for biochemical estimation. Since plasma is in equilibrium with extracellular fluid and hence, changes in plasma levels are more significant. Plasma and serum are interchangeable (except for fibrinogen studies, when plasma is used). It should be kept in mind that for some biochemicals including glucose, the blood values may be lower than plasma levels.

Since, it takes some time to separate plasma or serum from blood, therefore, the composition of blood may change during that period. Therefore, for components whose composition changes very rapidly, whole blood is preferred. These include pH, lactate, pyruvate and ammonia.

Blood is also used for determining glucose or urea, but plasma is preferable.

20. Which is more preferable serum or plasma for biochemical estimation?

Ans: Generally plasma and serum are interchangeable except for fibrinogen testing for which plasma is used. However, there are two factors that influence the choice.

a. If it is necessary to separate the cells immediately, then plasma is preferred because serum preparation needs 15–30 minutes of clotting.

b. If it is particularly important to avoid hemolysis because of leakage of enzymes from RBC into plasma, then serum is preferred. The reason is that it is easier to obtain 'hemolysis-free serum' than 'hemolysis-free plasma'. The possibility of having more chances of hemolysis in plasma is due to addition of anticoagulants such as citrates or oxalates. However, the hemolysis is less important with heparin and with special care.

21. How may the plasma proteins be precipitated?

Ans: The plasma proteins have isoelectric points between 4.9 and 7.6. At lower pH, these are present as cations and precipitated as insoluble salts of acids. Commonly used acids include tungstic acid, trichloroacetic acid.

At higher pH, the proteins exist as anions, therefore these are precipitated as insoluble salts with cations. The example includes alkaline zinc sulfate, cadmium sulfate and barium hydroxide.

22. What are the advantages of trichloroacetic acid over tungstic acid as protein precipitating agent?

Ans: Trichloroacetic acid gives more volume of filtrate from same volume of blood and filters more quickly than tungstic acid mixtures.

23. What are the different combinations of zinc salts used for protein precipitation?

Ans: a. *Zinc sulfate and sodium hydroxide*: It deproteinize whole blood, but fail to do with plasma.

  b. *Zinc sulfate and barium hydroxide*: It completely deproteinize whole blood, plasma and serum. It does not introduce any salt into the filtrate. It also precipitates anticoagulants such as oxalate and fluoride, if present in large amount.

24. What is the need of protein precipitation in biochemical analysis?

Ans: During biochemical analysis, there is a possibility of protein precipitation which will interfere with reading on spectrophotometer. Accordingly, sometimes it is desired that plasma proteins should be removed and deproteinated sample should be analyzed.

25. What is the limitation associated with deproteination of plasma samples?

Ans: The removal of proteins from blood/plasma may introduce many errors:

   a. Some of the components (that need to be determined) may also be precipitated with proteins.
   b. Some of the reagents used for protein precipitation may be incorporated in the sample that ultimately interferes with estimation.
   c. The dilution of plasma with protein precipitating agent may also influence the concentration of substance in the filtrates.

26. What are the biochemical techniques employed in which there is no need for protein removal?

Ans: The scientists have developed different techniques to avoid the need of deproteination of plasma. These include the need of:

   a. Use of greater dilutions at which proteins are not precipitated.
   b. Use of solubilizing agent to keep the proteins in solubilized form, e.g. use of p-toluene sulfonic acid and 2, 5-dimethyl benzene sulfonic acid.
   c. Use of high amount of urea also keep the denatured proteins in sample in solubilized form.
   d. Use of non-ionic surfactant such as Triton X-100, tween 20, etc.

27. What is the effect of hydrogen peroxide (a substrate) on catalase activity determination?

Ans: H_2O_2 is a substrate for catalase. However, it should be used only at lower concentration (about 10 mm). At higher conc., it damages the enzyme and hence, enzyme determination cannot be performed.

28. What are the different methods for quantitative determination of proteins?

Ans: a. Biuret method
   b. BCA (bicinchoninic acid) method
   c. Folin Lowry assay
   d. Bradford assay (Coomassie Brilliant Blue G-250)
   e. UV method
   f. Fluorimetric assay

29. What are the more sensitive methods for protein determination?

Ans: a. Biuret assay is not sensitive; therefore, proteins should be present in large amount. The sensitivity range is 0.1–0.8 mg.

b. BCA method is more sensitive than the biuret assay and proteins < 10 μg are measured.

c. Lowry method is one of the most sensitive protein quantification method and proteins in the range of 4–40 μg can be determined.

d. Bradford method is also a very sensitive method. The sensitivity range is 10–100 μg, but with micro-assay as little as 2 μg proteins can be determined.

30. What are the limitations of Lowry's method for protein determination?

Ans: a. The method is susceptible to various disturbances (even in low conc.) like EDTA, Sucrose, Glycine, Tris, detergent and inorganic salts including ammonium sulfate, sodium phosphate, sodium acetate.

b. A further disadvantage is that there is limited linearity of absorption upon increasing protein concentration. Therefore, it is necessary that the values of protein should lie within linear part of calibration curve.

31. What are the advantages and disadvantages of Bradford method over Lowry's method?

Ans: *Advantage*

a. Unlike Lowry's method, there is relatively little interference from substances like detergents.

Disadvantages

a. The major limitation of Bradford method is blue staining of cuvettes, therefore, disposable plastic cuvettes must be used. Glass cuvettes should be cleaned with acetone or incubated for several homes in 0.1 M HCl.

b. It does not measure accurately the complex protein mixtures. The reason is that binding of a dye to protein depends on the size and amino acid composition of protein. In complex mixture, there are all sorts of proteins, therefore, depending on the protein composition, different results are produced with this method.

c. Bradford assay is incompatible with surfactants at concentrations routinely used to solubilize membrane proteins. In general, the presence of a surfactant in the sample, even at low concentrations, causes precipitation of the reagent. Since the coomassie dye reagent is highly acidic, a small number of proteins cannot be assayed with this reagent due to their poor solubility in the acidic reagent.

32. What is UV method of protein determination?

Ans: The protein solutions exhibit absorbance at two wavelengths in UV region, at 210 and 280 nm. The absorbance at 280 nm is much stronger than at the corresponding of 210 nm. The absorbance at 280 nm is due to contribution of three aromatic amino acids, i.e. phenylalanine (257 nm), tyrosine (274.6 nm) and tryptophan (280 nm). The peak at 280 nm is dominated by tryptophan absorption peak.

Therefore, absorbance of a given protein solution is noted at 280 nm and from that absorbance, concentration of test solution of protein is calculated by comparing to standard protein solution.

33. What is the most sensitive method for protein determination?

Ans: The fluorimetric method assay is the most sensitive method and protein at the level of 0.5 μg can also be measured.

34. What do you understand by coupled reactions?

Ans: In quantitative biochemical analysis, in enzyme catalyzed reactions, either the appearance of product or disappearance of substrate is followed. However, sometimes there are no detectable changes between products and substrates. Therefore, it is a convenient method to couple a second or sometimes a third reaction to main (first) reaction to observe a reaction.

For example, determination of hexokinase activity

$$\text{D-glucose} + \text{ATP} \xrightarrow{\text{HK}} \text{glucose-6-P} + \text{ADP}$$

$$\text{Glucose-6-P} + \text{NADP}^+ \xrightarrow{\text{G6PDH}} \text{gluconate-6-P} + \text{NADPH} + \text{H}^+$$

In this first reaction, there is no detectable change. However, in second coupled reaction, NADPH is formed which can be detected at 340 nm.

35. Describe the differences between Lowry and Bradford methods of protein estimation.

Ans:

S. No.	Lowry's Method	Bradford's Method
1.	Lowry method is a colorimetric assay based on the interaction of protein with an alkaline copper tartrate solution and folin reagent. The color is generated by two steps: (1) formation of protein and copper complex in an alkaline buffer and (2) reduction reaction of folin reagent.	The Bradford assay is based on the association of specific amino acid residues, arginine, lysine, and histidine, with non-conjugated groups of Coomassie brilliant blue G-250 dye (CBB) in an acidic environment. The bindings of proteins with CBB result in a color change leading to a spectral shift.
2.	Lowry's modified assay is more sensitive.	Bradford assay is faster and a little less sensitive.
3.	Interfering substances include amino derivatives, ammonium sulfate, amino acids, buffers, detergents, EDTA, lipids, sugars as glucose and sucrose, nucleic acids several salts and phosphates, citrates, potassium and magnesium (ions that generally cause precipitation) ions.	Less interfering substances that include SDS, Triton X-100, commercial detergents, basic buffers, sodium hydroxide and Tris (> 2 M).
4.	It has main advantage that even complex mixtures of proteins may also be measured accurately.	It does not measure accurately the complex protein mixtures. The reason is that binding of a dye to protein depends on the size and amino acid composition of protein. In complex mixture, there are all sorts of proteins, therefore, depending on the protein composition; different results are produced with this method.

36. What is the principle of older methods of glucose determination in blood?

Ans: Before the introduction of glucose oxidase or o-toluidine methods, the most of methods employed for glucose determination included the following general procedure: Precipitation of blood proteins followed by reduction of alkaline cupric copper solution to cuprous oxide in the presence of glucose (reducing agent) or reduction of alkaline potassium ferricyanide to ferrocyanide (in the presence of glucose). These changes are associated with color development which is the basis of glucose determination.

37. What are the limitations of these older methods?

Ans: These older methods lack the specificity, i.e. other than glucose, other reducing agent present in the blood can also give the color reaction. The important reducing agent present in RBC is glutathione. Glucuronic acid is also present in appreciable quality that can also give reaction. Other component present in blood in small quantity includes urea, ascorbic acid and threonine.

38. What is the modification made in the above methods to overcome the problem associated with non-glucose reducing substances?

Ans: On addition of blood into an isotonic solution of sodium sulfate, in which cells are not hemolyzed, the diffusible substance move into the solution. The RBC which mainly contains non-glucose reducing substances are removed with protein precipitate (done with zinc sulfate and barium hydroxide).

39. What is the basic principle of glucose oxidase method of glucose determination?

Ans: The aldehyde group of glucose is oxidized by glucose oxidase to give gluconic acid and H_2O_2. H_2O_2 is broken down in the presence of peroxidase and oxygen acceptor to give a colored complex.

$$Glucose + H_2O_2 + O_2 \xrightarrow{\text{Glucose oxidase}} Gluconic\ acid + H_2O_2$$

$$H_2O + Oxygen\ acceptor \xrightarrow{\text{Peroxidase}} Colored$$
$$complex + H_2O + O_2$$

For example, oxygen acceptor is o-dianisidine. Nowadays, dianisidine (a carcinogenic agent) is replaced by a combination of phenol and 4-aminophenazone. H_2O_2 oxidizes phenol to give a substance which gives a colored product with 4-aminophenazone.

40. What are the factors that may influence the activity of glucose oxidase?

Ans: Presence of fluoride, protein precipitants, uric acid, glutathione and ascorbic acid influence the actions of enzyme.

41. What are the methods of glucose determination that give the true value of glucose?

Ans: Glucose oxidase methods and o-toluidine methods give the true value of glucose.

42. What is the principle of glucose estimation by o-toluidine method?

Ans: In this method, o-toluidine reacts with the terminal aldehyde group of glucose in the presence of hot glacial acetic acid to produce a blue-green colored condensation product that can be measured colorimetrically at λ of max 630 nm.

$$Glucose + o\text{-toluidine} \longrightarrow blue\text{-green complex}$$
$$(N\text{-glycosylamine})$$

43. What is the limitation of measuring glucose in blood after a long delay?

Ans: In a whole blood, glucose disappears very rapidly on standing. About 10 mg/ml may be lost per hour at room temperature due to conversion of glucose to lactose in a process of glycolysis. Therefore, determination of glucose after a delay gives lower value.

44. How is glycolysis prevented in blood?

Ans: Glycolysis can be prevented by adding sodium fluoride to the anticoagulant. A mixture of sodium fluoride and potassium oxalate in the proportion of 1 to 3 parts prevents the loss of glucose for two to three days. However, the excess should not be added as it interferes with estimation. Alternatively, the proteins may be precipitated from blood and removal of enzymes decreases the incidence of glycolysis. Glycolysis does not occur in plasma or serum.

45. Which is preferable for determining glucose among blood, plasma and serum?

Ans: The plasma is preferred over serum or blood. Between serum and blood, serum is preferred. Plasma is in equilibrium with extracellular fluid; therefore, plasma glucose levels more accurately reflect the glucose content of extracellular fluid.

46. Why plasma is preferred over blood for glucose determination?

Ans: The blood glucose concentration is always less as compared to plasma glucose (about 12–13%). Although the concentration of glucose in the water of cells and plasma is same, however, the water content in the cells (73%) is less as compared to plasma (93%). Therefore, the concentration of glucose is more in plasma than in blood.

47. What is the correction factor applied, if glucose is measured in blood?

Ans: The glucose content may be corrected by multiplying the whole blood glucose conc. by 1.15 and adding 0.33 mmol/l (6.0 mg/100 ml) to give plasma or serum glucose.

48. What is the effect of hematocrit in relation to closeness of blood glucose levels to plasma glucose levels?

Ans: Lower the hematocrit (in anemia), the more nearly to the whole blood glucose is to the plasma glucose, while for high hematocrit (polycythemia), the blood glucose levels are very different from the plasma glucose levels.

49. What are the advantages of plasma over serum in determining glucose levels?

Ans: a. Plasma has the advantage that blood can be directly added to a mixture of anticoagulant and can be separated immediately. Therefore, there are less chances of glycolysis during the brief period of plasma separation. In comparison, serum separation takes 15–30 minutes. Therefore, there are chances of glycolysis during this time.

b. More volume of plasma may be separated from same volume of blood than is obtained, if serum is separated.

50. What is the basic principle of Folin and Wu technique of glucose determination?

Ans: The method of Folin and Wu has been the most common method for blood glucose determination before the glucose oxidase add o-toluidine method. Glucose reduces the cupric ions present in the alkaline copper reagent to cuprous ions or the cupric sulfate is converted into cuprous oxide, which reduces the phosphomolybdic acid to phosphomolybdous acid, which is blue when optical density is measured at 420 nm.

51. What is the difference between arterial and venous blood glucose levels?

Ans: There is no difference between arterial and venous blood glucose levels at fasting level. However, when blood glucose levels are at peak (post prandial), the venous blood glucose is much lower than arterial blood glucose (20–35 mg/kg/100 ml). It is because of increased carbohydrate utilization at that time.

52. What is the renal threshold for glucose?

Ans: In normal persons, as long as the blood glucose is below 160–180 mg/100 ml, glucose is not excreted by kidneys in amounts as detected by route test. However, glucose starts appearing in urine, when the levels of glucose tend to increase above 180 mg/100 ml.

53. What is glucose tolerance test?

Ans: In order to measure the metabolic response of animal to glucose, the glucose tolerance test was devised. The test consists of giving specified amount of glucose and then testing the concentrations of glucose in the blood and urine at specific time intervals. This test establishes when the blood glucose reaches its highest concentration, when glucosuria occurs, and how rapidly the blood glucose concentration returns to normal.

54. What is the significance of glucose tolerance test?

Ans: a. It has importance in the investigation of symptomless glycosuria such as renal glycosuria.
b. These are also important in recognizing milder cases of diabetes.
c. However, it is rarely useful test in severe or established diabetes when the symptoms are almost quite definite.

55. What is the insulin tolerance test?

Ans: It is the test which is used to differentiate insulin resistant or insulin sensitive diabetes mellitus. In this test, insulin is injected intravenously in fasting conditions. The normal response is fall in approx. 50% of fasting glucose levels in about half an hour followed by rise back to normal fasting levels. In persons with insulin resistant diabetes, the fall in blood glucose is slight or negligible.

56. What do you mean by non-protein nitrogen (NPN)?

Ans: In blood, NPN means nitrogen from all nitrogenous substances other than protein. In urine (without protein), it is equal to total nitrogen. Urea is the most important substance of NPN. Others include uric acid, creatinine, creatine, amino acids and ammonia.

57. What is the principle of urea estimation by urease method using Berthelot reaction?

Ans: Urease specifically breaks down urea to form ammonia. Ammonia is allowed to react with phenol in the presence of hypochlorite to form indophenol which with alkali gives a blue colored compound. Nitroprusside acts as catalyst and also increases the intensity of color.

58. What is the principle of urea estimation by diacetyl monoxime method?

Ans: Urea reacts with diacetyl (a compound with two adjacent carbonyl groups) to give a colored compound. In fact, diacetyloxime is employed which decomposes to yield diacetyl and oxime. Diacetyl reacts with urea to give colored compound which is determined at 520 nm. In this method, thiosemicarbazide and ferric ions are added to catalyse the reaction.

59. Which is preferable serum/plasma or blood for urea determination?

Ans: The use of serum/plasma is preferable to whole blood.

60. How do the urea levels may decrease in the body?

Ans: The urea level over a period of time is proportional to protein content in diet. So its levels may be reduced due to poor protein content in diet.

61. What are the components in the body that converts to uric acid?

Ans: Uric acid is an end product of metabolism of purines including adenine and guanine.

62. What is the basic principle of uric acid determination?

Ans: Most of the methods used to determine uric acid are based on its reaction in alkaline solution with a phospho-tungstic acid reagent. In this reaction, uric acid is oxidized to allantoin and phosphotungustic acid to 'tungsten blue'.

63. What is the difference between creatine and creatinine?

Ans: Creatine is synthesized in liver and it is taken by skeletal muscles in which it is converted to creatine phosphate (energy rich source). On the other hand, creatinine is a waste product, which is excreted in urine. In a body, there is spontaneous conversion of creatine to creatinine about 2% per day.

64. What is the most common method of creatinine determination?

Ans: Creatinine is usually determined by Jaffe's reaction in which red color is produced on its reaction with alkaline picric acid. However, this reaction is not specific and other substances present in blood also give this color.

65. What is the role of nitric oxide in body?

Ans: Nitric oxide is a reactive radical gas that controls various vital physiological functions in the body. It plays a variety of roles such as maintenance of vascular tone, neurotransmission, and host defense by destroying microbes. Unregulated production of nitric oxide can cause nitrosative stress, leading to damage of proteins/DNA and to cell injury and death.

66. Why we choose nitrite/nitrate estimation as an index of NO production?

Ans: Nitric oxide (NO) is rapidly oxidized to nitrite and/or nitrate by oxygen. Integrated nitric oxide production can be estimated by determining the concentrations of nitrite and nitrate end products. The measurement of nitrate/nitrite concentration or of total nitrate and nitrite concentrations (NOx) is routinely used as an index of NO production.

67. What are the different methods to estimate nitric oxide?

Ans: There are different direct as well as indirect methods to measure nitric oxide production:

Direct methods: Chemiluminescence; Electrochemical; Mass spectral analysis

Indirect methods: Spectrophotometric determination using copper-cadmium alloy

68. How can copper-cadmium alloy be prepared?

Ans: Copper is mixed with cadmium by melting these two metals in a crucible. The molten alloy is made into a block immediately, which is thereafter converted to powder using a metal file.

69. What ratio of copper is used to prepare cadmium alloy and why?

Ans: The addition of 10% copper to cadmium is preferred as this ratio shows the maximum conversion efficiency. Higher ratios of copper (15% and 20%) in the cadmium alloy results in the development of a blue color during nitrate reduction, which subsequently interferes with the final color development by the Griess reagent.

70. What is the major concern to keep in mind during spectrophotometric determination of serum nitrite and nitrate by copper-cadmium alloy?

Ans: The nitrite concentration in the samples should be determined without addition of the alloy, while the nitrite plus nitrate concentration is determined in the presence of the alloy.

71. What is the principle of spectrophotometric determination of serum nitrite and nitrate by copper-cadmium alloy method?

Ans: It is the most commonly used indirect method for spectrophotometric determination of serum nitrite and nitrate (indirectly nitric oxide). The principle of the assay is the reduction of nitrate by copper-cadmium alloy followed by color development with Griess reagent (sulfanilamide and N-naphthylethylenediamine) in acidic medium.

72. What are the advantages and disadvantages of using cadmium alloy over other methods to measure nitric oxide?

Ans: *Advantages*

a. It is a single step method used to measure nitrate/nitrite in serum and plasma.
b. Rapid and inexpensive
c. The copper-cadmium alloy used in the present method is easy to prepare and can completely reduce nitrate to nitrite in an hour
d. These alloy fillings can be stored for 2–3 months at 2–8 °C after activation. They are required in very small quantities.

Disadvantages

a. Nitrate reduction by cadmium is difficult because it must be activated every time and used immediately.
b. Amount of cadmium required for each assay is also relatively high.

73. What are the different methods of deproteination in nitric oxide estimation?

Ans: a. Somagyi reagent
b. Carrez reagent

74. What is Griess reagent?

Ans: It is sulfanilamide and N-naphthylethylenediamine used for color development on reaction with nitrite/nitrate.

75. What is Somagyi reagent?

Ans: It is zinc sulfate and sodium hydroxide used to deproteinize the sample.

76. What is Carrez reagent?

Ans: It is zinc acetate and potassium ferrocyanide used to deproteinize the sample.

77. What is the principle of superoxide dismutase assay by epinephrine autoxidation method?

Ans: Epinephrine undergoes autoxidation in the presence of EDTA and sodium carbonate at pH—10.2 to give adrenochrome which is detected at 480 nm. However, in the presence of superoxide dismutase, the autoxidation of epinephrine to yield adrenochrome is prevented. Therefore, the ability of dismutase to inhibit the autoxidation of epinephrine is the basis of its assay.

Biostatistics

8

1. Describe importance of statistics in pharmacology.

Ans: Statistics is an important tool in pharmacological research that is used to summarize experimental data in terms of central tendency (mean or median) and variance (standard deviation, standard error of the mean, confidence interval or range). More importantly, it enables us to conduct hypothesis testing and make conclusion based on the results.

2. Discuss applications of statistics in pharmacology.

Ans: Statistical applications in pharmacology include in bioequivalence, bioavailability, drug discovery and toxicological studies. Statistics can be very helpful in formulating experimental design and drawing appropriate inferences (conclusions) from the collected data.

3. What are the most common descriptive statistics used in biological system?

Ans: 'Mean' and 'standard deviation' are two of the most common descriptive studies for continuous data.

4. What is the limitation of using these descriptive statistics?

Ans: These statistics describe correctly only for normal or Gaussian distribution of values. However, for non-normal distribution, these relationships are not valid, so mean and standard deviation should not be used. Instead median and range are more recommended. It is also noteworthy that most of biological data are not normally distributed.

5. What do you understand by the term variable?

Ans: A variable is any characteristics, number, or quantity that can be measured or counted.

6. Classify different variables.

Ans:

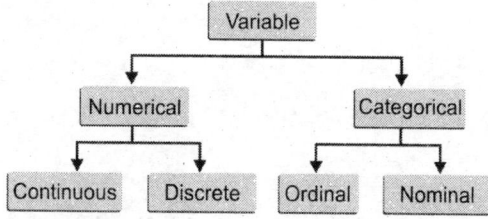

7. Differentiate numerical and categorical variables.

Ans: *Numerical variable* describes a measurable quantity as a number, like how much/how many. The data collected for numerical value is *Quantitative data*.

Categorical variable describes a 'quality' or 'characteristic' of a data unit, like 'what type' or 'which category'. The data collected is called *Qualitative data*.

8. Differentiate between discrete and continuous variables.

Ans: *Discrete variables* are those in which there are possible numbers of outcomes. Observations can take a certain value based on a count. For example: Number of animals that die when 12 animals have been tested for LD_{50}.

Continuous variables are those in which there is unlimited number of possible outcomes in some interval. Observations can take any value between a certain set of real numbers. For example: Weight of animal can have any value between 180 and 220.

9. Differentiate between ordinal and nominal variables.

Ans: *Ordinal variables* are those in which observations can take a value that can be logically ordered or ranked. The categories associated with ordinal variables can be ranked higher or lower than another. For example: Effect of drug may come under ordinal data by ranking the effects low, medium and high.

Nominal variables are also called categorical variables. These are variables in which observations can take a value that is not able to be organized in a logical sequence. A purely categorical variable is one which can be assigned to categories, but cannot be ranked in a sequence. For example: Gender is a categorical variable having two categories (male and female) and these cannot be ranked in any order.

10. What are different types of averages?

Ans: Mean, median and mode are different types of averages.

11. Define mean.

Ans: This is also called the arithmetic mean. The sample mean is computed as the sum of all the observed outcomes (X) divided by the total number of events (N).

12. Define median.

Ans: The middle value of a sample is called median. The median depends on whether the number of observations is even or odd. If the number of terms is odd, then the median is the value of the term in the middle. If the number of terms is even, then the median is the average of the two terms in the middle.

If the number of terms is odd, i.e. 3, 5, 7, 9 and 11, then median is 7 (middle one).

If the number of terms is even, i.e. 3, 5, 7, 9, 10 and 11, then median is 8 (average of 7 and 9, two middle terms).

13. What is mode?

Ans: The mode of a distribution is the value that occurs most often or most frequently. The mode of a data is the number with the highest frequency. For example: 8, 10, 10, 100, 200 is a set of numbers. The number 10 recurs most often and considered as mode.

14. What are the different ways of representing the variation in a numerical data?

Ans: The variation is represented by various ways that may include range, variance, standard deviation, coefficient of variation and standard error of mean.

15. Define range.

Ans: It is the difference between maximum and minimum values in a data.

16. What do you understand by the term variance?

Ans: The variance is a measure of how far each value in a data is from the mean value. The higher value of variance indicates that individual values are very different from mean values. On the other hand, small variance indicates that individual values are very near to mean value and are not very different from it.

The sample variance is denoted by (σ^2).

$\sigma^2 = \Sigma [(x_i - \bar{x})^2]/n - 1$.

$\bar{x}$ is mean and x_i is individual value, n = number of observations.

17. What do you mean by standard deviation (SD)?

Ans: It is another way of representing the variation in a data and tells us how much variation we can expect in a population. It is the square root of the variance and denoted by σ.

18. What is the advantage of representing the variability of data in standard deviation than variance?

Ans: Standard deviation is usually more useful to describe the variability of the data while the variance is usually much more useful mathematically. Though the value of variance is theoretically correct, it is difficult to apply in a real world sense because the values used to calculate it are squared. Advantages of standard deviation over variance are as follows:

- Standard deviation, as the square root of the variance, gives a value that is in the same units as the original values. So, standard deviation has the convenience of being expressed in units of the original variable.
- It is easier to work with and easier to interpret in conjunction with the concept of the normal curve.

19. Explain the significance of standard deviation.

Ans: In a normal, symmetric and bell-shaped distribution, about two-thirds (about 66.67%) of the individual values are between +1 and −1 standard deviations from the mean. Furthermore, standard deviation is approximately 1/4th of the range in small samples (N < 30) and 1/5 to 1/6 of the range in large samples (N > 100).

20. Explain the above described significance of standard deviation with suitable example.

Ans: If a mean value of a given data is 50 for 100 observations and standard deviation is 7, then 66.67 values shall lie between 43 and 57 (between +1 and −1 standard deviations from the mean).

Furthermore, if highest value of a data is 70 and lowest value is 30, then range of a data is 40. Since, standard deviation is about 1/5th to 1/6th of the range (for 100 or more observations), therefore, the value of standard deviation should be between 6.6 and 8. It is an approximate method to calculate the standard deviation without using a formula.

21. What is standard error mean (SEM)?

Ans: Standard error of mean quantifies the extent to which the process of sampling has misestimated the population mean. Standard error of mean is a type of standard deviation which describes the accuracy of sample mean with respect to population mean. Smaller the standard error, the greater the certainty with which the sample mean estimates the population mean.

22. Differentiate between SD and SEM.

Ans: Standard deviation (SD) is a measure of dispersion of the original random variables within sample, whereas standard error (SEM) is the measure of dispersion (variation) of sample mean from a population mean. SD quantifies how much the values show a discrepancy from one another within a sample, whereas SEM quantifies how precise is the sample mean and how much it differs from true mean of the population.

SD gives the dispersion of batch and SEM gives the dispersion of population.

23. **What is the coefficient of variation or relative standard deviation (RSD)?**

Ans: It is another way of representing the variation of a data and is the ratio of the standard deviation(s) to the mean (μ).

Coefficient of variation (CV) = σ/μ

24. **What are the different types of CV?**

Ans: There are inter-assay CV and intra-assay CV, Generally, intra-assay % CV should be less than 10 and inter-assay % CV should be less than 15. Experimental results with poor intra-assay CV (> 10%, more than 10%) frequently reflect poor pipetting technique.

25. **What are commonly used statistical methods for assay validation?**

Ans: The commonly used statistical methods for assay validation include:

a. *Regression analysis*: Particularly with respect to accuracy, linearity, limit of detection and limit of quantification

b. *Analysis of variance (ANOVA)*: Particularly with respect to reproducibility of assay under a variety of test conditions such as different laboratories, assay temperature and days

26. **What is the difference between accuracy and precision?**

Ans: *Accuracy* is the degree of conformity of a measured or calculated quantity to its actual (true) value. The accuracy of an experiment is a measure of how closely the experimental results agree with a true or actual value.

On the other hand, *precision* is a measure of reproducibility of an experiment. It is the degree to which further measurements/calculations show the same/similar results. In other words, the precision of an experiment is a measure of the reliability of the experiment (Fig. 8.1).

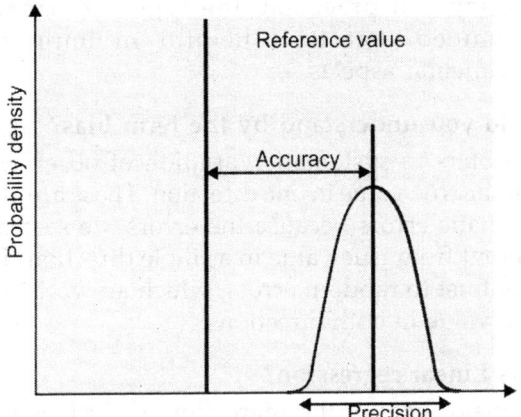

Fig. 8.1: Representation of accuracy and precision

27. **Explain the difference between accuracy and precision with suitable example.**

Ans: Accuracy is the degree of closeness to true value, whereas the precision is degree to which an experiment will repeat the same value. For example, the true or reference value is 15 and in experiments performed by A and B, the values comes out to be 12 and 14. In this case, the experiment performed by B is more accurate. On repetition of same experiment, if values of A and B again comes out to be 12 and 13, then experiment of A is more precise, though inaccurate. The experiment of B will be less precise, though accurate.

Therefore, it is not necessary that precision and accuracy coexist. An experiment may be accurate, but not precise and vice versa can also coexist. However, it is always desirable to have both precision and accuracy in experiments.

28. **What is the significance of accuracy and precision in making conclusions regarding the errors in experiments?**

Ans: Both accuracy and precision are measure of error in experiments. An inaccurate value may be due to personal error or instrumental error. However, lack of precision indicates the personal error. Therefore, from accuracy and precision, the types of error may be determined that it is helpful in improving the experimental aspects.

29. What do you understand by the term bias?

Ans: Bias refers to systematic variation of observed values from the true value in one direction. These are also called systematic errors because the errors are systematically different from true value in a single direction. These are in contrast to random errors, which are variations from mean value in both directions.

30. What is Linear regression?

Ans: The major goal of the regression analysis is to predict the values. It is a method of estimating/predicting a value of dependent variable provided the values of independent variables are known. It is based on the principle of association/relationship between dependent and independent variables. For example: Health of a person (dependent variable) may be predicted by age, body weight, and disease (independent variables).

31. What are the basic types of regression analysis?

Ans: There are two basic types of regression analysis: Simple regression and multiple regression. In simple regression, the value of dependent variable is predicted using a single independent variable. On the other hand, in multiple regression, the value of dependent variable is predicted using a number of independent variables. The above described example of predicting the health on the basis of age, body weight, medical history and disease is a type of multiple regression.

32. What is symmetric distribution?

Ans: Distribution that has the same shape on both sides of the center is called symmetric. A symmetric distribution with only one peak is referred to as a normal distribution.

33. What is binomial distribution?

Ans: The binomial distribution is applicable for the following conditions:

a. For n observations, there is possibility of only one of two outcomes; one is typically called a success and the other failure.
b. The probability of a success, p, is the same from observation to observation.
c. Each observation is independent of the others.

34. What is discrete random variable distribution?

Ans: It is another name of binomial distribution. It is named so because in the binomial distribution, probability of observing x number of successes out of n observations is always discrete (countable) and random.

35. What is normal distribution?

Ans: The normal distribution is a continuous random variable distribution and it is represented by a normal density curve (Fig. 8.2).

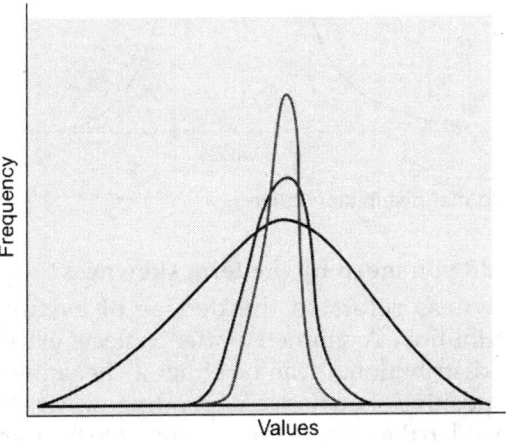

Fig. 8.2: Different normal distribution curves same mean but with different standard deviations

36. What do the mean and standard deviation specify in a normal distribution curve?

Ans: The mean specifies the location of distribution and the highest point of the normal curve is termed the mean of the population.

Standard deviation specifies the spread of the distribution. Furthermore, the shape of the curve is influenced by the standard deviation, i.e. for higher standard deviation, the shape is broad, and for narrow standard deviation, the shape is narrow. Three normal density curves with the same mean (location), but different standard deviations (spreads) (Fig. 8.3).

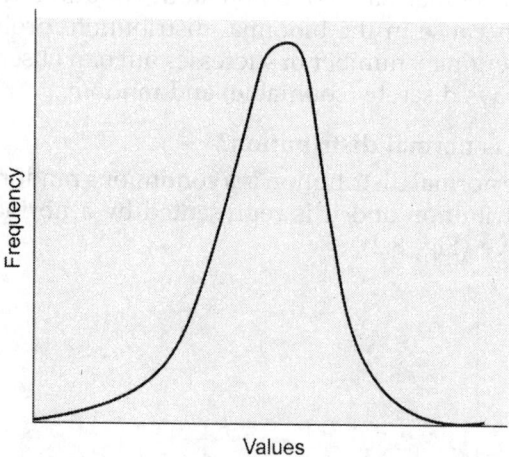

Fig. 8.3: Normal distribution curve

37. What do you mean by the term skewness?

Ans: Skewness refers to the degree of asymmetry in a distribution. Asymmetry often reflects extreme values in a distribution. It can be either a "negative skewness" or "positive skewness", depending on whether data is skewed to the left (negative skew) or to the right (positive skew) of the data average.

38. Describe various types of skewness.

Ans: *Positively skewed*: A distribution is positively skewed when it has a tail extending out to the right. In positively skewed distribution (Fig. 8.4):
   a. Mean is greater than the median.
   b. Mean is sensitive to each value in the distribution.
   c. It is subject to large shifts when the sample is small and contains extreme values.

Negatively skewed: A negatively skewed distribution has an extended tail pointing to the left. It is more or less similar to positive skewed distribution in various characteristics, except that median is larger than mean (Fig. 8.4).

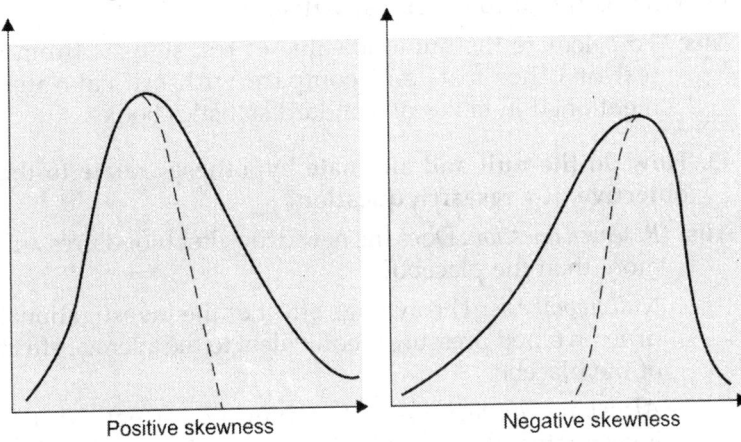

Positive skewness   Negative skewness

Fig. 8.4: Representation of positive and negative skewnesses

39. What do you mean by hypothesis testing?

Ans: Hypothesis testing is a statistical method in which an appropriate statistical test is used to make a decision, i.e. accept or reject a hypothesis. In drug testing, a decision is made whether a drug is efficacious or not at a particular dose level.

40. What are the different steps of hypothesis testing?

Ans: The hypothesis testing involves number of steps including:

   a. Formulating a null hypothesis
   b. Formulating an alternative hypothesis
   c. Deciding an appropriate statistic test to be applied
   d. Deciding the critical value depending on a probability
   e. Calculating the numeric value of test statistic (say t-test or ANOVA)
   f. Comparing the test statistic value with critical value
   g. Accepting or rejecting the null hypothesis.

41. What is critical value? How is it calculated?

Ans: It is defined by choice of 'α' and type of distribution. It is the value which is used to reject or accept null hypothesis. It is seen from statistical tables given in books.

42. What is the purpose of test statistic?

Ans: To calculate the numeric value of test statistic (from t test or other test) and compare with critical value mentioned in tables of standard statistics books.

43. How do the null and alternate hypotheses relate to the objective of a research question?

Ans: *Research question*: Does the new drug alter blood pressure more than the placebo?

Null hypothesis: The average effect of the investigational drug on blood pressure is equivalent to the average effect of the placebo.

Alternate hypothesis: The average effect of the investigational drug on blood pressure is not equivalent to the average effect of the placebo on blood pressure.

44. What do you mean by probability or *p-value*?

Ans: The *p-value* is the probability of rejecting or accepting the null hypothesis (H_0) of a study question. It determines the significance or non-significance of results.

The probability of something happening can be expressed using any number from 0 to 1. A probability of 0 means the event will never happen. A probability of 1 indicates that an event will always happen. A probability of 1/3 signifies that the event has a 1 in 3 chances of occurring.

- A small *p-value* (typically < 0.05) indicates strong evidence against the null hypothesis, so the null hypothesis is rejected. It means investigational drug is different from placebo.
- A large *p-value* (> 0.05) indicates weak evidence against the null hypothesis, so the null hypothesis is not rejected. In this case, investigational drug is not different from placebo.

45. What is the limitation of the *p-value*?

Ans: Limitation of the *p-value* is that it may be influenced by study results. It also does not show the magnitude of difference between the groups.

46. When does a non-significant *p-value* occur?

Ans: A non-significant *p-value* (large *p-value*) may occur because of either:

a. there are no differences between the two study groups, i.e. two means are almost similar.

b. The study does not have sufficient 'control' to show a difference between the two study groups, i.e. when sample size is much smaller. However, with sufficiently large sample sizes, the power of test may be increased and statistical difference may be obtained.

47. What is the significance of alpha (a design parameter)?

Ans: The α (alpha) is a part of study design and is generally fixed to 0.05 (means 95% confidence level). By using α, the critical region is calculated from table. Thereafter, test statistic value is compared with critical region (so hypothesis is accepted or rejected). However, the values of α may also be changed to 0.1 (90% confidence level) or 0.01 (99% confidence level).

48. In statistics, what does alpha (α) indicate?

Ans: α is the probability of making a type I error. Higher the confidence level, lesser is the probability of making an error. For example, at 95 % confidence level, the chances of making a type I error is 0.05, while it reduces to just 0.01 at confidence level of 99%.

49. What is the difference between α and *p-value*?

Ans: Generally, these are used interchangeably. However, these two are different. α is a 'study design' and its value is fixed at the time of formulating hypothesis (0.05–0.1). However, *p-value* is experimental outcome. After applying approximate test, a *p-value* comes and is helpful in accepting or rejecting null hypothesis.

50. How to interpret *p-value* with α?

Ans: The following is a helpful way to interpret *p-value*:
  a. Hypothesis is rejected, if the calculated *p-value* ≤ α, i.e. *p* is less than fixed 0.05.
  b. Hypothesis is not rejected, if the calculated *p-value* ≥ α, i.e. *p* is greater than fixed 0.05.

51. What is level of significance?

Ans: The person conducting the hypothesis test specifies the maximum allowable probability of making a type I error (hypothesis true but test rejects it), called the level of significance for the test. It is expressed in percentage (%), i.e. 5% or 1%. It is the confidence with which the experimenter rejects or retains the null hypothesis. For example: At 5% level of significance, the person has 5% chances of making wrong decision and making type I error.

52. What is confidence limit/interval?

Ans: A term used in statistics that measures the probability that a population parameter will fall between two set values. The confidence interval can take any number of probabilities, with the most common being 95% or 99% among 99%, 98%, 95% and 90%. The z value for a 95% confidence interval is 1.96.

$x \pm z_{a/2} \times \sigma / \sqrt{(n)}$.

x, represents the mean.

53. What are the different components of confidence interval?

Ans: There are three components:
  a. Point estimate: Is actually a sample mean which represents the best estimate of the population mean.
  b. Standard error
  c. Reliability factor

54. How do confidence intervals may be determined on the basis of mean and standard error?

Ans: Confidence intervals may be determined as exemplified by following values:

Confidence intervals (CI) = Sample mean ± SE × Reliability factor

Let us assume mean of 100 values (sample mean) is 62.6 and SE is 1.20. At different confidence levels (90 %, 95 % and 99 %), the intervals are:

- At 90% confidence level, CI = 62.6 ± (1.20)(1.66) = (60.6, 64.6)
- At 95% confidence level, CI = 62.6 ± (1.20)(1.98) = (60.2, 65.0)
- At 99% confidence level, CI = 62.6 ± (1.20)(2.63) = (59.4, 65.8)

55. What is the statistical interpretation of above exemplified confidence intervals?

Ans: A statistical interpretation of these results is that, we are 90% confident that the mean value of the population is enclosed in the interval 60.6–64.6. If greater confidence is required (with 99% confidence), the mean value of population is enclosed in the interval 59.4–65.8. It can be clearly seen that for higher confidence level, the confidence interval is higher indicating the more unreliability.

56. What do confidence intervals indicate?

Ans: A sample drawn from a large population is used to calculate an average or a mean value. However, sample mean is not a population mean. However, on the basis of sample mean, confidence intervals are calculated that serve as an estimate for unknown fixed value of population mean. In the above example, the sample mean is 62.6, however, there is a probability that population mean may range between 59.4 and 65.8 at 99% confidence levels.

57. What is reliability factor?

Ans: It is used to quantify how close our estimate (calculated mean) is to be the real population mean.

58. On what factors, the reliability factor depends and how is it determined?

Ans: The reliability factor depends on value of alpha (α) and degree of freedom (sample size).

Its value is noted from the table given in standard statistical books on the basis of alpha (α) and degree of freedom. For example, for a sample size 100 (99 degree of freedom), the reliability factor for two sided 90%, 95% and 99% confidence levels are 1.66, 1.98 and 2.63, respectively. The higher value of reliability factor indicates less reliability.

59. What is the implication of reliability factor with respect to confidence levels?

Ans: The more value of reliability factor at higher confidence level indicates that, if higher confidence is required, the estimate becomes less reliable. On the other hand, at low confidence levels, the estimate becomes more reliable.

60. What is the difference between *p-value* and confidence interval?

Ans: The important difference between the *p-value* and confidence interval is that the confidence interval represents the clinical significance, whereas *p-value* indicates statistical significance. Therefore, the confidence interval is mostly preferred in clinical study instead of *p-value*.

61. What is degree of freedom?

Ans: It is calculated as the difference between the number of observations or sample size n and the number of parameters estimated. Degree of freedom denotes the number of samples that a statistician has the freedom to choose.

If number of parameter = 1,

sample size = 30;

Then, the degree of freedom = 30 – 1 = 29

62. What do you mean by type I and type II errors?

Ans: *Type I error:* It occurs when null hypothesis is actually true, but is rejected as false by testing. It is denoted by α-error (false positive). In type I error (or false positive), there is no difference between two means, but by error it is accepted that these two means are different.

Type II error: It occurs when null hypothesis is actually false, but is accepted as true by testing. It is denoted by β-error (false negative). It means that two means are actually different, but by error actually it is assumed that these are same.

63. Which is more dangerous type I or type II error?

Ans: Both the errors are dangerous, but type II error is more dangerous, particularly in drug development. In type I error, an error is made by assuming that investigational drug is different from placebo. However, there are chances of making the correction during subsequent steps of drug testing. It means even if a non-active drug is falsely accepted as active drug, it will be rectified during subsequent steps of drug development.

However, during type II error, an error is made by assuming that investigational (active) drug is not different from placebo. In other words, an active drug is rejected considering it as inactive drug. This is very dangerous as this error cannot be corrected in subsequent steps of drug development because the active drug is already being rejected in initial steps of drug evaluation.

64. What do type I and type II errors indicate in clinical trials?

Ans: In a clinical trial, type I error is committed when we claim that a new drug is superior to placebo, while in reality they are same.

Type II error is committed when we fail to claim that a new drug is superior to placebo, while in reality they are different.

65. Classify biostatistical tests.

Ans: For analyzing different types of data, statistical tests are mainly divided into two groups.

    a. *Parametric tests*: These tests are used for normal distribution of data. Examples include: Unpaired student t-test, paired t-test, one way ANOVA, repeated measures ANOVA, and Pearson correlation coefficient.

b. *Non-parametric tests*:

   I. These tests are used when data is not normally distributed.

   II. These methods are most appropriate when the sample sizes are small. When the data set is large (e.g. n > 100) it often makes a little sense to use nonparametric statistics at all.

   III. It is also used for non-numeric value (ordinal) Example: Chi-square test, Fischer's test, Mann-Whitney U test, Wilcoxon signed rank test, Friedman's test and Spearman rank order.

66. What are the requirements for applying parametric test?

Ans: Parametric test can be applied to data:

a. which is normally distributed.

b. which is numerical in nature.

c. which observations are independent in a group.

67. What are the requirements for non-parametric test?

Ans: Parametric test can be applied to data:

a. which is non-normally distributed.

b. which is of ordinal type (non-numeric).

c. which observations within group are independent.

68. What are the advantages of non-parametric test?

Ans: The non-parametric or distribution free methods are popular in the analysis of biological data because of the following:

a. It is simpler to use without much mathematical calculations.

b. Unlike in the t test, no assumption is made regarding the nature of the distribution so that the test can be applied irrespective of the data being normally distributed.

69. What are the factors on which selection of a test is based?

Ans: The selection of the appropriate test is based on the:

a. Nature of the experiment

b. Type of questions to be answered

c. Types of variable being analyzed

70. What is student's t-test? Why is it called so?

Ans: Student's t-test is used for assessing the statistical difference between two sample means.

Student's t-test was introduced by William Sealy Gosset, a statistician working in Dublin in 1908. His employer, Guinness Breweries, allowed him to publish his findings under a pseudo-name, which he chose as "Student". Therefore, the test that he described is known as 'Student t-test'.

71. What are the conditions for using student's t-test?

Ans: In general, t-test requires two independent variables (an experimental and a control group) and a single continuous dependent variable. It may be used in the following conditions:

a. to calculate statistical significance between two samples.

b. when sample size is 30 or less and population standard deviation is not unknown.

72. What are paired and unpaired t-tests?

Ans: Depending on the types of sample, student's t-test is of two types: Paired and unpaired t-tests.

Paired t-test (Dependent t-test) is used to compare means of two dependent samples. It is used to compare the pre-treatment and post-treatment groups within a same animal. For example, in rota rod experiment, the effect of muscle relaxant is analysed by comparing the pre-treatment and post-treatment readings in a same animal.

Unpaired t-test (Independent t-test) is used to compare means of two independent samples, i.e. to compare control and treatment groups as different animal groups. In this case, control and treatment groups constitute different animal groups, which in contrast to previous case, in which each animal served as control as well as treatment. For example, in pentylenetetrazole induced convulsion experiments, the effect of anti-epileptic drug is analyzed using two different animals, control (in which no drug is given) and treatment (in which drug is given).

73. Differentiate between paired and unpaired t-tests.

Ans:

	Unpaired t-test	Paired t-test
a.	Two independent groups are compared.	Two dependent groups are compared.
b.	Intragroup variability is present because control and treatment groups constitute two different animal groups.	No intragroup variability is present, because control and treatment groups constitute same animal group.
c.	More animals are required because control and treatment groups are performed animals.	Lesser number of animals are required because in different control and treatment groups may be performed in same animal.

74. What is the disadvantage of paired t-test?

Ans: A disadvantage of the paired design test is that it takes a lot of time to complete the experiment. The reason is that readings have to be taken for pre-treatment and post-treatment groups in same animal. On the contrary, in unpaired t-test, the readings are taken concurrently in separate animals, which make an experiment much shorter in duration.

75. What do you understand by term ANOVA?

Ans: ANOVA means analysis of variance. Despite its name, ANOVA works by comparing the difference between means of different groups, rather than the difference of variance between different groups. In ANOVA, variance between different groups is calculated and is used to determine whether the means are different or not.

76. What are the different steps using which ANOVA can be applied on samples?

Ans: 1. ANOVA partitions the total variability in the experiment (the total sum of squares) into components (sums of squares) due to 'between treatment' and 'within treatment' variabilities.

2. Both of sums of squares are then divided by the appropriate degrees of freedom to yield a 'mean square between groups' and a 'mean square within groups'.

3. 'mean square within groups' is an average of the variances within groups and is a measure of biological variability.

4. Ratio of the 'mean square between groups' to the 'mean square within groups' is the 'F-statistic' or' F-ratio', a measure of differences among groups.

5. If there are no real differences among the groups, the value of the F-statistic should be close to 1.0.

6. If the F-value is larger than the appropriate critical value (which depends on the degrees of freedom), it is concluded that the observed differences are not due to chance alone and state that the differences are statistically significant.

77. What is the major difference between ANOVA and t-test?

Ans: In a t-test, two sample means are compared with each other to find any statistical difference. ANOVA is the extension of t-test. However, the major difference between the ANOVA and t-test is that, ANOVA is used to compare the means between more than two groups.

78. When is analysis of variance applied?

Ans: Analysis of variance is used to compare three or more groups with quantitative variable. It tells that if one of the group means is different from the other means. If there is a single/one independent variable, then it is a one-factor (way) ANOVA; while for two independent variables, two-factor (way) ANOVA is used.

79. What do you understand by ANOVA between group and within group?

Ans: There are two types of ANOVA that can be used for a statistical model of a particular research hypothesis. 'Between groups ANOVA' is appropriate to use when hypothesis involves more than two groups with different participants in each group and each group receives different treatments. For example: Participants in different groups are subjected to different treatments to determine the effect of medication on disease state. Thereafter, the results of different groups are compared by applying 'between group ANOVA' to make a conclusion whether there is any statistical difference between effect of different drugs on disease.

80. What do you understand by 'ANOVA within group'?

Ans: 'ANOVA within group' is also called 'one way repeated measure ANOVA.' It is used when a single drug/ treatment is given and responses are noted on different time intervals/days. In this case, the aim is to determine the statistical difference between the effects of a single drug on a same animal on different times. It is called ·repeated measure because the same responses are repeatedly measured in a single group with same treatment.

81. What are the different types of ANOVA?

Ans: a. *One-way ANOVA between groups*: This type of ANOVA is used to compare the difference between different groups.

b. *One-way repeated measure ANOVA (One-way ANOVA within group)*: A one way repeated measure ANOVA is used when a single drug/treatment is given and responses are noted on different time intervals/days.

c. *Two-way ANOVA between groups*: A 'two-way ANOVA between groups' is used to compare the statistical difference between different groups on different time intervals or some other variable such as gender.

d. *Two-way repeated measure ANOVA*: In this type of ANOVA, same animal is subjected to more than one treatment and response is noted at different time intervals.

82. What are the advantages of using two-way ANOVA?

Ans: 1. *Interaction*: Two-way ANOVA allows to consider interaction, i.e. if there is an interaction between the two independent variables on the dependent variable. It allows to get a more accurate representation of how the response variable depends on the two factors.

2. *Fewer type II errors*: Two-way ANOVA considers more sources of variability than each individual one-way ANOVA does. Therefore, there are fewer type II errors during statistical testing.

83. What is the limitation of using t-test to compare more than two sample mean?

Ans: Using independent t-test to compare more than two sample means instead of ANOVA may produce more type I errors (reject null hypothesis, when it is true). For example: If t-test is to be applied for comparing four means for statistical difference, at 0.05 significance level, then 6 independent t-tests have to be conducted. During this process, the probability of not committing a type I error decreases significantly from 0.95.

Furthermore, it is very complicated to apply 6 independent t-tests to compare four means as compared to applying a single ANOVA.

84. What do you understand by two-way repeated measure ANOVA?

Ans: In this ANOVA, same animal is subjected to more than one treatment and response is noted at different time intervals. It is called "two-way" because there are two factors in the experiment. For example, different treatments and time intervals. The word 'repeated-measure' is used because same response is measured repeatedly on the same subject on different time intervals.

85. What do you understand by two-way ANOVA between groups?

Ans: A 'two-way ANOVA between groups' is used to compare the statistical difference between different groups on different time intervals or some other variable such as gender. The primary purpose of a two-way ANOVA is to understand, if there is an interaction between the two independent variables (such as treatment and time/gender) on the dependent variable (response).

86. Differentiate between one-way ANOVA and two-way ANOVA.

Ans: One-way ANOVA test is able to assess only the effect of different treatments at a given time. Two-way ANOVA, on the other hand, evaluates the effect of both time and treatment on a given response. Furthermore, it also evaluates whether there is an interaction between variables such as time and treatment parameters. A two-way test generates three *p-values*, one for each variable independently, and one measuring the interaction between the two variables.

87. What is post hoc test? Why is it used?

Ans: It is a test which is applied after applying ANOVA. ANOVA tells us that there are differences between the groups. However, it is unable to tell which group is different from others. Therefore, after applying ANOVA, more specialized test (post hoc test) is applied to find the difference among the different groups.

88. What are different post hoc tests?

Ans: Dunnett's test, Bonferroni test, Scheffe's test, Fisher's LSD and Tukey's range test.

89. What are the advantages of Bonferroni's test?

Ans: Bonferroni's method has the main advantage that it maintains an overall type I error. It is a very conservative test, therefore, the chances that null hypothesis is rejected, when it is not, is very less. It is conservative because the critical values required for rejection are very large as compared to other tests.

90. What is the significance of Tukey's test? How is it different from Dunnett's test?

Ans: Tukey's test is a multiple comparison test in which pairwise comparison is made between all groups. In other words, all the groups are compared with one another.

On the other hand, in Dunnett's test, a comparison is not made between all the groups. Rather, all the groups are compared with one a single group, i.e. control group. In other words, this test is used for comparing all groups with a control group.

91. What is Chi-square test (X^2)?

Ans: A Chi-square (X^2) statistic is employed to test the difference between an actual sample and previously established distribution such as which may be expected due to chance or probability.

92. What is Fischer exact test? Why is it so called?

Ans: Fisher's exact test was invented by English scientist Ronald Fisher, and it is called exact because it calculates statistical significance exactly, rather than by using an approximation. Fischer exact test is used to evaluate the statistical significant difference between groups possessing categorical data (qualitative data). It is one of the number of tests used to analyze contingency tables, which display the interaction of two or more variables. It is applied to less sample size (< 5 samples).

93. What is the major difference between the Chi-square and Fischer exact tests?

Ans: Fischer's exact test is a way to test the association between two categorical variables when the sample size is small (less than 5). Chi-square test is used when the sample size is large.

94. What is Mann-Whitney U test?

Ans: This test is performed when data of two groups is qualitative in nature and is ranked on an ordinal scale. Furthermore, this test is applied to large sample size (n > 100). It is a very useful test as it has high power approximately 95% compared to unpaired t-test. The principle in applying the Mann-Whitney U test is to rank the data in an order and different groups are compared with one another on the basis of their rank totals.

95. What is Wilcoxon signed-rank test?

Ans: This is the non-parametric test and is analogues to the parametric paired t-test. It should be used, if the distribution of differences between pairs is not normally distributed. Wilcoxon signed-rank test is used when there are two nominal variables and one measurement variable. One of the nominal variables has only two values, such as "before" and "after," and the other nominal variable often represents individuals.

Hence, the group has no difference if,

Sum of positive ranks = Sum of the negative ranks

96. What is the difference between Mann-Whitney U test and Wilcoxon signed-rank test?

Ans: Both these test are non-parametric tests. Mann-Whitney U test is analogous to unpaired t-test, whereas Wilcoxon signed-rank test is analogous to the paired t-test.

97. What are the disadvantages of Mann-Whitney U test and Wilcoxon signed-rank test?

Ans: Both tests are based on comparison between medians and do not refer to means. The major limitation is that even if there is no significant difference between groups, even then it cannot be concluded that samples are the same.

98. Name the software used in the Biostatistics.

Ans: There are several softwares used in the Biostatistics. Most commonly used softwares are SPSS, Sigma plot, Graph Pad prism, Instat, Biostat and Statistica.

Ethical Issues in Experimental Pharmacology

9

FOR UNDERGRADUATES AND POSTGRADUATES

1. What do you understand by CPCSEA?

Ans: CPCSEA stands for Committee for the Purpose of Control and Supervision of Experiments on Animals.

2. What is the goal of CPCSEA guidelines?

Ans: The goal of these guidelines is:

   a. to promote the humane care of the animals used in biomedical and behavioral research.
   b. to perform testing with the basic objective of providing specifications that will enhance animal well-being quality in the pursuit of advancement of biological knowledge that is relevant to humans and animals.

3. What do you understand by quarantine?

Ans: Quarantine is the separation of newly received animals from those already in the facility until the health and possibly the microbial status of the newly received animals have been determined. An effective quarantine minimizes the chances for introduction of pathogens into established colony.

4. What is the duration of quarantine for laboratory animals?

Ans: A minimum duration of quarantine for small laboratory animal is one week and a larger animal is 6 weeks (cat, dog and monkey).

5. **Why quarantine method is used in laboratory?**

Ans: a. Effective quarantine procedure is used for non-human primates to help limit exposure of human zoonotic infection.

b. Physical separation of animals by species is recommended to prevent interspecies disease transmission and to eliminate anxiety and possible physiological and behavioral changes due to interspecies conflict.

c. It shall be acceptable to house different species, in same room, e.g. if two species have a similar pathogen status and are behaviorally compatible.

6. **How can transgenic animals are acquired?**

Ans: These animals can be either developed in the laboratory or produced for R & D purpose from registered scientific/academic institutions or commercial firms and generally from abroad with approval from appropriate authorities.

7. **What are special precautions for maintaining transgenic animals?**

Ans: The transgenic and knock-out animals should be maintained in clean room environment or in animal isolators. These animals carry additional genes or lack of genes compared to the wild population. To avoid the spread of the genes in wild population care should be taken to ensure that these are not inadvertently released in the wild to prevent cross breeding with other animals.

8. **What are the important guidelines for the use of restraint equipment?**

Ans: The following are the important guidelines for the use of restraint equipment:

a. Restraint devices cannot be used simply for convenience in handling or managing animals.

b. The period of restraint should not be the minimum requirement to accomplish the research objectives.

c. Animals to be placed in restraint devices should be given training to adapt to the equipment.

9. **What are the effective environmental parameters should be followed for laboratory animals?**

Ans: Temperature and humidity controls prevent variations due to changing in climatic conditions or differences in the number and kind of room occupants.

   a. Ideally, capability should be provided to allow variations within the range of approximately 18 to 29 °C (64 to 84.2 °F), which includes the temperature range usually recommended for common laboratory animals.

   b. The relative humidity should be controllable within the range of 30 to 70% throughout the year. For larger animal, a comfortable zone (18 to 37 °C) should be maintained during extreme summer by appropriate methods for cooling.

10. **What do you understand by 3Rs principle?**

Ans: To achieve the significant difference or hypothesis, 3Rs should be followed which can be described as:

   a. *Replacement*: If possible, replace the methods in animals with *in vitro* or in silico methods.

   b. *Refinement*: To minimize potential pain, suffering or distress to animal used during experiments

   c. *Reduction*: If not possible to select any other *in vitro* procedure, then minimize the number of animals used for experimentation.

11. **When and why pre-anesthetic anesthesia is necessary?**

Ans: Before using actual anesthetics for surgery, the animals are prepared for anesthesia by overnight fasting and using pre-anesthetics agents, which reduce parasympathetic stimulation of cardiopulmonary system and reduce salivary secretion. Atropine is the most commonly used anticholinergic agent.

12. **What are the CPCSEA guidelines for surgery in animals?**

Ans: Multiple surgical procedures on a single animal for any testing or experiment are not to be practiced unless specified in a protocol only approved by the IAEC.

13. **What is the maximum experimentation period for an animal?**

Ans: Animal should not be subjected to experimentation for more than 3 years.

14. **What is the guideline regarding use of neuromuscular blockers?**

Ans: Neuromuscular blocking agents must not be used without adequate general anesthesia.

15. **How does animal should be prepared before induction of anesthetic?**

Ans: Before using actual anesthesia, the animal is prepared for anesthesia by overnight fasting and using pre-anaesthetic, which blocks parasympathetic stimulation of cardiopulmonary system and reduce salivary secretion. Atropine is the most commonly used anticholinergic agent.

16. **What are the ethical issues associated with blood collection technique from retro-orbital sinus?**

Ans: This method is controversial because it produces discomfort to animals. Inflammation reactions are produced at the site of puncture (visualized after 4 days). Mostly, these reactions tend to heal after 4 weeks. However, there may be a possibility of formation of hematoma in retro-orbital site. The pressure of hematoma may compress the optic nerve to produce blindness.

17. **What are the general criteria for euthanasia?**

Ans: The method should in all cases meet the requirements:
   a. Death, without causing anxiety, pain or distress with minimum time lag phase
   b. Minimum physiological and psychological disturbances
   c. Compatibility with the purpose of study and minimum emotional effect on the operator

BIBLIOGRAPHY

1. A method to perform direct transcutaneous intrathecal injection in rats. Mestre C, Pélissier T, Fialip J, Wilcox G, Eschalier A. *J Pharmacol Toxicol Methods*, 1994; 32:197–200.

2. A method to perform direct transcutaneous intrathecal injection in rats. Mestre C1, Pélissier T, Fialip J, Wilcox G, Eschalier A. *J Pharmacol Toxicol Methods* 1994 Dec; 32(4): 197–200.

3. Biological Effects of Blood Loss: Implications for sampling volumes and techniques. McGuill MW, Rowan AN. ILAR News, 1989; 31: 5–20.

4. Biostatical analysis 4th edition, 1999. Jerrold H. Published by Dorling Kindersley Pvt. Ltd.

5. Biostatistical analysis 4th edition, 2007. Zar JH. Published by Pearson Education.

6. Drug Bioscreening: Drug evaluation techniques in pharmacology, 1990. Emmanuel B. Thompson. VSH Publisher, USA.

7. Drug transport in brain via the cerebrospinal fluid. Fluids Barriers CNS. 2011 Jan 18;8(1):7. Pardridge WM. doi: 10.1186/2045-8118-8-7.

8. Essentials of Medical Pharmacology, 6th edition, 2013. Tripathi KD. Published by Jaypee Brothers Medical Publishers Pvt. Ltd.

9. Evaluation of Drug Activites: Pharmacometrics Vol 2, 1964. Laurence DR and Bacharach AL, Academic Press, London and New York.

10. Fundamentals of Experimental Pharmacology, 4th edition, 2008. Ghosh MN. Published by Ghosh SK, et al. 109, College Street, Kolkata-12, 37.

11. Guidelines for the Survival Bleeding of Mice and Rats, 2010: oacu.od.nih.gov/ARAC/documents/Rodent_Bleeding.pdf

12. Handbook of Experimental Pharmacology, 3rd edition, 2009. Kulkarni SK. Published by Vallabh Prakashan, Delhi.

13. Measurement of Nitric Oxide Production in Biological Systems by Using Griess Reaction Assay. Sun J, Zhang X, Broderick M and Fein H, *Sensors* 2003; 3:276–84.

14. Methods in Drug Evaluation: Proceedings of the Intranational Symposium held in Milano, 20–23 September 1965. Editors— Mantegazza P and Piccinini F, North Holland Publishing Company, Amsterdam.

15. Pain and Analgesia in Domestic Animals: Handbook of Experimental Pharmacology; Livingston A 2010; (199):159–89.

16. Practical Clinical Biochemistry: General topics and commoner tests, 5th Edition. Varley Harold, Gowenlock Alan H, Bell Maurice. William Heinemann Medical Books Ltd, 1980; 1192–3.

17. Practical Enzymology 2nd edition, 2004. Hans Bisswanger. Published by Wiley VCH Verlag GmbH & Co. KGA.

18. Practical Manual of Experimental and Clinical Pharmacology, 2010. Medhi Bikash. Published by Jaypee Brothers Medical Publisher Pvt. Ltd.

19. Principles of Neuropsychopharmacology, 1997. Feldman RS, Meyer JS, Quenzer LF. Published by Sinauer Associtaes, Inc., Publishers.

20. Remington: The Science and Practice of Pharmacy, 20th edition, volume 1, Lippincott Williams and Williams, 2000.

21. Short Protocols in Pharmacology and Drug Discovery: A compendium of methods from current protocols in pharmacology. Edited by: Enna SJ, Williams Michael, Ferkany John W, Kenakin Terry, Porsolt Royer D. Published by: John Wiley & Sons, Hoboken, New Jersey.

22. Spectrophotometric determination of serum nitrite and nitrate by copper-cadmium alloy. Sastry KV1, Moudgal RP, Mohan J, Tyagi JS, Rao GS. *Anal Biochem* 2002 Jul 1;306(1):79–82.

Index